Integrative Strategies
for Cancer Patients

A practical resource for managing
the side effects of cancer therapy

Integrative Strategies for Cancer Patients

A practical resource for managing the side effects of cancer therapy

Written by internationally renowned leaders in integrative medicine at **Columbia University Medical Center, New York**

Elena J. Ladas, MS, RD
Kara M. Kelly, MD
Columbia University, USA

Contributing Authors : Christine Grimaldi, PhD, Deborah Hughes Ndao, MPH, Diane Rooney, MS, LAc, LMT, and Katherine Taromina, MS, LAc

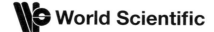

NEW JERSEY · LONDON · SINGAPORE · BEIJING · SHANGHAI · HONG KONG · TAIPEI · CHENNAI

Published by

World Scientific Publishing Co. Pte. Ltd.

5 Toh Tuck Link, Singapore 596224

USA office: 27 Warren Street, Suite 401-402, Hackensack, NJ 07601

UK office: 57 Shelton Street, Covent Garden, London WC2H 9HE

British Library Cataloguing-in-Publication Data
A catalogue record for this book is available from the British Library.

INTEGRATIVE STRATEGIES FOR CANCER PATIENTS
A Practical Resource for Managing the Side Effects of Cancer Therapy

ISBN-13 978-981-4313-23-0 (pbk)
ISBN-10 981-4313-23-8 (pbk)

Typeset by Stallion Press
Email: enquiries@stallionpress.com

Printed in Singapore by Mainland Press Pte Ltd.

"As an hematologist and oncologist, researcher, and pioneer in the field of integrative oncology, I have witnessed how patients value the use of integrative therapies in managing the side effects of cancer therapy. *Integrative Strategies for Cancer Patients* is an easy to follow hands-on guide for patients, their caregivers and practitioners. Ladas and Kelly demonstrate the role of integrative therapies in cancer care, and most importantly, build on evidence based research. I strongly recommend this book for guidance on strategies for symptom management in cancer care."

David Rosenthal, MD
Professor of Medicine, Harvard Medical School
Medical Director, Zakim Center for Integrative Therapies
Dana-Farber Cancer Institute
Director, Harvard University Health Services

"Rarely does a book fulfill the promise of its title as well as this invaluable volume. Ladas and Kelly provide a gift to people living with cancer — this wealth of information that will serve to empower them through the use of complementary therapies to maximize their quality of life. Definitely added to my recommended reading list!"

Donald I. Abrams, MD
Integrative Oncology
UCSF Osher Center for Integrative Medicine

"I was a cancer patient more than 25 years ago. Faced with little hope, I turned to alternative medicine and cured myself. How I wish a book like this had existed then so I had understood my options. This work beautifully blends conventional and complementary wisdom, resulting in the most comprehensive and compassionate care we can imagine. An invaluable tool to practitioners, patients and families, it weaves all the options together into a tapestry of healing that will best serve the patient in their recovery."

Christina Pirello
Emmy Award winning host of the national public television series, 'Christina Cooks'
Bestselling author
Cancer survivor

"I was 28 years old and had just started my intern year as a pediatric resident, when I was diagnosed with a rare condition affecting mostly children. I was treated at the Herbert Irving Comprehensive Child and Adolescent Oncology Center at Columbia University Medical Center and underwent 6 months of chemotherapy, one life changing experience, that would have been unbearable if it wasn't for the help I received by the integrative medicine team. Yoga, nutrition counseling and cooking classes, herbal remedies, reiki, aromatherapy, acupuncture helped me tremendously with the side effects I suffered. I learned a lot, as a human being, but also as a physician. My pediatric clinic offers all the wonderful therapies that made such a difference in my life. I have experienced the benefits of these therapies firsthand and because of this, I can highly recommend *Integrative Strategies for Cancer Patients*. This book is a rich resource for anyone, of any age, battling cancer."

Anja Widmann, MD
Clinica Oasis del Pacifico
Puerto Escondido, Mexico

"Coming from a family that unfortunately has cancer thread throughout the generations, the value of this book is limitless both mentally, physically, and soulfully. The importance of how to find ways to cope, not only as a patient, but also as a survivor, healing practitioner, and caregiver, with cancer side effects that will help to bring back some living of life and relief during these times. Through these integrative therapies you will find some positive peace within and with people around you, which will then hopefully radiate to some better outer well being and healing during this challenging journey. This is a true revolutionary new way of added caring treatment for cancer coming from the heart!"

Elisabeth Halfpapp
Exhale executive, VP Movement Programming
New York City

"My cancer diagnosis and ensuing chemotherapy and radiation left me feeling lethargic, weak, and above all, powerless. Through working with the recommendations highlighted by *Integrative Strategies for Cancer Patients*, I learned about the links between diet and illness, and I have since radically altered my lifestyle. Three years later I am cancer-free and have never felt healthier or more energetic! This book has the potential to empower cancer patients to take control of their health and overcome the daunting obstacles they face."

Chloe Greenbaum
Cancer Survivor
New York

ALL PROCEEDS FROM THE SALE OF THIS BOOK WILL BENEFIT
THE INTEGRATIVE THERAPIES PROGRAM FOR CHILDREN
WITH CANCER

For all adults, adolescents, and children battling cancer

Acknowledgements

We would like to thank the many individuals who helped make this book possible. Foremost, Sid and Helaine Lerner have provided unrelenting support for the vision of The Integrative Therapies Program for Children with Cancer. Dr Michael Weiner, Hettinger Professor of Clinical Pediatrics Director, Herbert Irving Child and Adolescent Oncology Center at Columbia University Medical Center, Morgan Stanley Children's Hospital of New York, for his leadership and support in enabling us to develop the first comprehensive pediatric integrative oncology program. We applaud the dedication and support of the physicians of Columbia University Medical Center. With gratitude, we thank Evelyn Li, LMT, LAc for her expert review of the aromatherapy sections of the manuscript, Barbara McClenahan for her editorial expertise on early drafts of the book, and Alanna Cabrero for her dedication to the field of integrative oncology. We would like to thank Julie Mosow for her editorial guidance. We are grateful to our publisher, World Scientific Publishing Company Pte Ltd, for supporting the development of this project.

We especially want to thank our patients and their families who have been our greatest teachers. For all those who have allowed us to share in their joy and in their sorrow, and to learn lessons with them on their journeys through cancer treatment. We would like to especially acknowledge Bonnie Rogers, Jody and Sarah Scheinfeld, Josued and Sujelin Disla, Killian Mansfield and family who provided guidance on the text and layout of the handbook.

Finally, thank you to our families and friends who supported us in our endeavor in bringing this book to the public.

Contents

Contents

Chapter 1

The Role of Complementary Medicine and Cancer Treatment

With a diagnosis of cancer comes the need to make decisions about many different types of therapies. **Conventional therapies** are the treatments, including surgery, radiotherapy, chemotherapy, hormonal and biological therapies, that doctors use as part of medical care to treat people with cancer. These treatments are usually tested using scientific reasoning and research methods to demonstrate their benefits and evaluate their possible side effects.

Many patients wish to consider other ways to fight their cancer or manage the side effects of conventional therapies. **Complementary and alternative medical therapies (CAM)** are therapies that are frequently considered by patients that have been diagnosed with cancer. **Complementary and alternative medical therapies** are defined as a group of diverse medical and health care systems, practices, and products that are not presently considered to be part of conventional medicine. Other names for CAM include "natural," "holistic," "home remedy," "folk medicine," "Eastern medicine," or "unorthodox."

More specifically, **complementary therapies** are CAM therapies that are used along with conventional therapies, generally for management of symptoms related to the cancer or its treatment. Examples include acupuncture for cancer-related pain or ginger supplements for chemotherapy associated nausea. Use of complementary therapies by patients with cancer is generally more acceptable to doctors, although many doctors do not routinely recommend complementary therapies because many of these treatments have not yet been scientifically tested in large trials by conventional medical researchers.

Alternative therapies are CAM therapies that are used in place of conventional therapies, as a specific treatment for the cancer. Examples include special diets or dietary supplements for treatment of cancer. People try alternative therapies for many different reasons. Some are frightened by the possibility of unpleasant side effects from conventional therapies, such as chemotherapy or radiotherapy. Others believe that conventional therapies won't be beneficial. Some are misled by claims from alternative medicine practitioners of cancer cures. The benefits of alternative treatments are unproven — most alternative therapies have not been adequately tested, and to date, research studies have not shown that they can cure cancer or slow its growth. Like some conventional therapies, alternative therapies can also cause severe side effects, some of which may even be life threatening. There is also concern that some alternative therapies may interfere with the beneficial effects of conventional therapies if taken together.

People living with cancer and their caregivers may be very vulnerable to the claims of success often attributed to alternative therapies. Some alternative practitioners may take advantage of these emotions and promise miraculous cures, leading to a sense of false hope. Some alternative therapies are marketed in such a way that they seem to be very effective for treating cancer and yet have few side effects. Most alternative therapies are not reimbursed by commercial or government insurance programs (since they have often not been scientifically tested); consequently these therapies may be very expensive for the patient.

A preferred approach is one that incorporates **integrative medicine**. Integrative medicine is a comprehensive approach to healthcare that incorporates the mind, body and spirit, through the use of conventional therapies and those complementary therapies that have shown the greatest benefits. Integrative medicine provides benefits for coping with the side effects, managing the stress related to the diagnosis of cancer and its treatment, and helps the patient and caregiver to feel in control. The therapies highlighted in this book emphasize those therapies that may be effectively used in an integrative approach along with conventional therapies during and after the cancer experience.

The National Center for Complementary and Alternative Medicine (NCCAM) at the US National Institute of Health was established in 1998 with its mission to investigate CAM therapies in the context of rigorous science and to disseminate reputable information on CAM therapies to the public and professional communities. Proven treatments, often called "evidence-based," are therapies that have been tested following a strict set of guidelines and found to be safe and useful. Research results are published in peer-reviewed journals, where the articles are studied by other doctors or scientists in the field to be sure that they meet certain standards. Patient testimonials and marketing brochures do not meet these standards for evidence.

Experts at NCCAM have classified CAM therapies into five main categories. The therapies recommended in this book fall within most of these categories:

- **Mind–Body Medicine–** Practices based on the belief that your mind is able to affect your body.
  - o Yoga
  - o Visual Imagery
  - o Aromatherapy
- **Biologically Based Practices–** Therapies derived from nature.
  - o Aromatherapy
  - o Nutrition
  - o Herbal Teas
  - o Supplements
- **Manipulative and Body–Based Practices–** Therapies that involve manipulation of one or more parts of the body.
  - o Massage
  - o Reflexology
- **Energy Medicine–** Practices based on the belief that the body has energy fields that can be used for healing and wellness.

- **Whole Medical Systems**- Healing systems and beliefs that have evolved over time in different cultures and parts of the world.
  o Ayurvedic Medicine: Yoga, Herbal Medicine
  o Traditional Chinese Medicine: Acupressure, Tui Na, Nutrition
  o Homeopathy

Some medical centers provide integrative oncology services so that patients may receive complementary therapies alongside the conventional therapies. In some places, these programs provide a mechanism to advance scientific knowledge and clinical practice in the field of integrative oncology. Integrative oncology centers vary considerably in the comprehensiveness of the services they offer. Examples of services offered include acupuncture, massage, nutrition and supplement counseling, and mindfulness based meditation training for stress management. The resource section in this book provides information on how to identify credible integrative practitioners. A major advantage of receiving care at an integrative oncology center is that it often facilitates communication between your doctors and the practitioners providing complementary services.

Cancer and the conventional therapies used to treat it are associated with a wide range of side effects. Unfortunately, conventional therapies do not always adequately manage these side effects. Some side effects are easily controlled, whereas others require specialized management. Combinations of therapies, or varying the approaches, may be more effective in controlling the symptoms over the course of the cancer treatment experience. In conventional medicine, one therapy may work well for one patient and not so well for another. This also holds true for complementary therapies in cancer care.

Self help measures and therapies that can be administered by caregivers, such as the therapies highlighted in this book will hopefully yield a more comprehensive approach for treating the mind, body and spirit. We encourage you to experiment with the different therapies presented in this book, in order to identify the most effective approaches for symptom management during and after cancer therapy.

If you are considering using complementary or alternative therapies, talk to your doctor for advice and support. Doctors will generally support the use of complementary therapies to assist with coping during and after cancer treatment, and usually advise against using alternative therapies.

Chapter 2

Communicating with Your Medical Team

Good communication with your medical team is essential during cancer treatment. Open dialogue with the members of your conventional medical team including nurses, nurse practitioners, nutritionists, physician assistants, and doctors is an important part of understanding and coping with all phases of conventional cancer treatment. Not only does good communication build trust between you and your medical team, but it also facilitates the sharing of information between all of your medical providers and caregivers.

Ideally your doctor or nurse practitioner and complementary medicine practitioner would communicate with each other directly. However, in practice this is often difficult to achieve, and you may need to serve as an intermediary. Sometimes your conventional medical team may not have enough knowledge about a complementary medicine therapy and may rely on limited evidence-based research to help you make a decision. Your complementary medicine practitioner may also have limited information about your conventional diagnosis; including the cancer and the prescribed treatment. By opening the lines of communication, you are encouraging the professionals involved in your care to obtain information to ultimately meet your needs and improve your overall well-being during cancer treatment. Open communication facilitates your doctor's involvement in your decision-making about complementary medicine, and may allow your complementary medicine practitioner to have a more integrated and informed role in developing your treatment plan. With this approach, you too will feel more in control over your health.

Tips for Talking with Your Medical Team

• Prior to your visit: List the complementary medicine therapies you are interested in and the reasons you would like to use them. If possible, include documentation from a credible website or scientific journal about the use of the therapy in the setting of cancer. Suggested resources for information on complementary therapies may be found in Appendix I.

• On any patient history intake forms: Be sure to list any complementary medicine therapies you have used in the past during your cancer treatment, are using now, or are considering using during cancer treatment.

• Communicate openly: Speak to your medical team any time you are considering a complementary medicine therapy.

• Discuss with your doctor: Ask your doctor to review what is known about the safety, effectiveness and any potential or known interactions of the therapy of interest. Understand that your doctor may not have expertise in this area but can help direct you to credible resources, or may work with you in identifying credible resources for information.

• Enable communication: Provide the contact information for your complementary medicine practitioner. Request that correspondence be sent with details of your conventional therapy plan.

Tips for Talking with Your Complementary Medicine Practitioner

- Prior to your visit: Make a list of the components of your cancer treatment. For example, write down the chemotherapy drugs you will be receiving. Also, note any potential side effects related to your conventional cancer therapy.
- On any patient history intake forms: Be sure to list any conventional therapies you are using now, or are considering using for treatment of your cancer. Include other conventional medications prescribed along with your cancer treatment, such as medications to prevent nausea or antibiotics to reduce the risk of an infection. Describe any physical limitations you have.
- Speak to your complementary practitioner: Ask about his or her qualifications, where he or she learned about the particular complementary medicine specialty, and his or her experience working with other patients that share your particular health condition and concern. Ask the complementary practitioner about his or her experience in working in conjunction with conventional medical teams.
- Discuss limitations: Ask if you should adapt the complementary medicine therapy for any physical limitations you may have. Ask your complementary practitioner if there are any limitations of the therapy.
- Discuss interactions: If your provider is recommending nutrition or herbal supplements, ask about the evidence supporting the supplements and if they could interact with your conventional medical plan.
- Open communication between those involved in your medical care: Provide your complementary medicine practitioner with the contact information of your doctor. Ask that correspondence be sent with details of your complementary therapy plan.

What To Do If Your Doctor is Dismissive

- Discuss potential alternatives with your doctor. Have you found evidence to support the use of the complementary therapy for the side effect of interest? If not, could you substitute another complementary therapy that is supported by evidence?
- Investigate the interests of collaborating doctors within your medical center. Determine if a doctor within your medical group has received education or training in complementary therapies. For example, some medical doctors also are trained as licensed acupuncturist. Is there a doctor involved in research in complementary therapies?
- Contact a center with an integrative medicine program. Request an integrative consultation, and include your doctor in this consultation. If your doctor is unable to attend, request a comprehensive summary of your visit be sent to your oncologist.
- Contact experts in the field of integrative medicine. Both adult and pediatric cancer research networks have doctors who conduct research in complementary therapies. Contact these researchers. New research may be available on the therapy of interest.

• Review the information provided by the National Cancer Institute's (www.cancer.gov), Office of Cancer Complementary/Alternative Medicine (www.occam.gov/cam/), and the National Institute of Health's Center for Complementary and Alternative Medicine (www.nccam.nih.gov). You may be eligible to participate in a clinical trial investigating a therapy of interest (www.clinical trials.gov).

Chapter 3
How To Use This Book

This book is designed to serve as a practical guide for integrative care, the combination of both complementary medicine therapies and conventional medicine during cancer treatment. It does not have to be read from cover to cover, but instead is designed to be used as a reference resource. Common side effects experienced by people undergoing treatment for cancer are covered. Before referring to a specific chapter, it is important to review Chapter 4. This chapter provides specific details on the techniques and contraindications associated with each of the complementary medicine therapies presented in this book. For management of specific side effects, you can then refer to the corresponding chapters.

The goal of this book is to provide considerations on how to incorporate complementary medicine therapies in the management of side effects associated with cancer treatment. The complementary medicine therapies covered in this book are ones that can be *self-administered* or *administered with the assistance of a caregiver*. For some conditions, we suggest consultation with a licensed professional such as an acupuncturist. The therapies include: Aromatherapy, Chinese medicine and Acupressure, Herbal Teas, Homeopathy, Massage, Nutrition, Reflexology, Supplements (Nutrition, Herbal), Visual Imagery, and Yoga. For each side effect, only the therapies that the authors believe may be beneficial are presented in alphabetical order.

Each chapter reviews both the conventional medicine and Chinese medicine perspectives, and the integrative approach for its management. Integrative Medicine in Action (Patient Story) highlights those therapies that we most frequently rely on for the side effect and are based upon actual clinical cases. If a specific complementary therapy is not a therapy that is routinely applied for the given side effect, the therapy is omitted. The Appendix provides illustrated descriptions of acupressure point instruction, muscle reference model, reflexology foot and hand charts, yoga instruction, nutrition reference materials, references, and resources.

Sample Side Effect Chapter

What is <Side Effect>?

Provides the medical overview of the side effect, including the medical definition and causes.

How is <Side Effect> Treated by Conventional Medicine?

Provides the conventional treatments for the side effect.

Integrative Approaches to <Side Effect>

Presents the integrative approaches for the side effect. Provides considerations for choosing and applying complementary therapies.

Integrative Medicine in Action (Patient Story)

Patient stories present actual clinical cases that combine conventional medicine and complementary therapies. These are presented to serve as a guide for integration into medical care.

Aromatherapy

Suggested aromatic oils and applications are presented for the side effect. Aromatherapy application instructions are described in Chapter 4.

Chinese Medicine/ Acupressure

A Chinese medicine perspective of the condition and associated acupressure points are provided. Location of the points is located in Appendix A. Application of acupressure is described in Chapter 4.

Herbal Teas

Loose leaf teas and dosing guidelines are suggested for the side effect. Direction on the preparation and storage of tea can be found in Chapter 4.

Homeopathy

Commonly used homeopathic remedies and dosing guidelines are provided for the side effect. Details of homeopathy and potential risks and benefits are described in Chapter 4.

Massage

A massage sequence self-administered or delivered by a caregiver is pictorially demonstrated for each side effect. Muscle descriptions and locations can be found in Appendix B. Massage application instructions are described in Chapter 4.

Nutrition

Foods, beverages, and spices are provided for the side effect. Main nutrition strategies for each side effect highlighted under "quick dietary tips".

Reflexology

Foot and hand points are pictorially presented for each side effect. Reflexology application instructions can be found in the Introduction. Complete reflexology charts are located in Appendix C.

Supplements

Nutrition or herbal supplements and dosing guidelines are provided within the chapter for each side effect. Considerations for the use of supplements are provided in Chapter 4.

Visual Imagery

Guided imagery instruction is specified.

Yoga

Postures (asanas) and breathing exercises (pranayama) are listed. Instructions can be found in Appendix D. Information on postures, breathing, and cautions with yoga may be found in Chapter 4.

Chapter 4
Descriptions of Complementary Medicine Therapies

Rather than providing a comprehensive list of all available complementary medicine therapies, in this book, we present complementary medicine therapies which we have found to be beneficial in supporting patients with cancer. The complementary medicine therapies included here are: Aromatherapy, Chinese Medicine and Acupressure, Herbal Teas, Homeopathy, Massage, Nutrition, Reflexology, Supplements (Nutrition, Herbal), Visual Imagery, and Yoga. We selected these particular therapies based on our extensive expertise in working with adults and children undergoing treatment for cancer. Specific therapy recommendations are based on supporting scientific research and historical use, along with our clinical experience. Therapies with scientific evidence supporting their benefit in cancer care are especially highlighted. There may be other complementary therapies not covered in this book that could also be beneficial. If you are interested in obtaining further information on additional therapies, refer to Appendix I.

Brief overviews of each of the complementary medicine therapies are presented in this chapter. You will also find a list of important precautions associated with each of the complementary medicine therapies.

Aromatherapy

Aromatherapy is the use of essential oils for healing purposes. Dating back several thousand years, aromatherapy is easy for people of all ages undergoing cancer treatment to use. Essential oils are liquids extracted from flowers, herbs, and trees. The characteristic odor and healing benefits of each essential oil comes from its chemical composition. Essential oils can tone, stimulate, calm or balance, depending on their chemical makeup. In this book, we recommend 100% essential oils to ensure the purity and quality of oil.

We recommend specific aromatic oils as part of a fundamental aromatherapy kit or "starter" kit for beginners of aromatherapy. We suggest you begin with: Black pepper (*Piper nigrum*), Cypress (*Cupressus sempervirens*), Frankincense (*Boswellia carteri*), Ginger (*Zingiber officinale*), Lavender (*Lavandula angustifolia*), Lemon (*Citrus x limon*), Orange (*Citrus sinensis*), Peppermint (*Menthe piperita*), and Roman chamomile (*Matricaria recutita*). This collection of essential oils can be used for all of the side effects covered in this book. Essential oils can be applied by inhalation, topically through the skin, or orally by ingestion.

Inhalation (Breathing) Applications

Inhaling essential oils is the oldest, fastest, and simplest way to introduce essential oils into your body. Based upon your preference, essential oils can be inhaled by different methods.

Bowl and Towel: Add 2 to 6 drops of essential oil in a bowl of hot water. Place a towel over your head and keeping your eyes closed, lean over the bowl and inhale and exhale deeply.

Diffusion: Diffusers dispense essential oils into the air using electricity. Cold air diffusers and electrical fan diffusers disperse essential oils into the air without heating or burning and are optimal for use. Diffuse an essential oil for 15 to 30 minutes by sprinkling 3 to 6 drops of essential oil on a diffuser pad. Avoid diffusing essential oils by a heat-driven source, such as with candles.

Direct Inhalation: Directly inhale using a tissue sprinkled with 2 to 4 drops of an essential oil or inhale directly from the bottle. If inhaling directly from the bottle, be sure to wave the bottle under the nose about 1/2 inch from your nostril. For a stronger scent, move the bottle closer to your nose, as tolerated.

Mist: Add 8 to 10 drops of essential oil to a 4 ounce mister bottle or pump bottle filled with distilled water. Shake vigorously before use and spray in room or on skin.

Topical Applications (Applied to Body)

Topical applications of essential oils can be given in a bath, a compress, or diluted in carrier oil. Carrier oils are cold pressed vegetable oils, such as almond, grapeseed, sesame, peanut, and olive oil. Experiment with different applications to discover which works best for you. Be aware that skin irritation may develop after exposure to certain essential oils. Before beginning, we recommend that you do a patch test using double the concentration of the essential oil you would like to use. For example, if you were going to use one drop of lavender essential oil use two drops of the oil for the patch test. To perform a patch test, place the concentrated form of the essential oil on an adhesive bandage and apply to the skin for 6 to 12 hours. Once you remove the bandage, check the area for skin itching, redness or any other skin discomfort. If you do not experience any irritation, you may proceed to use this essential oil.

Most topical aromatherapy applications should be used with a two percent dilution. This means that for every two drops of essential oil, 98 drops of carrier oil should be used or for every 10 to 12 drops of essential oil 1 ounce of carrier oil should be used. Below are some suggested topical applications:

Bath: Dissolve 5 to 10 drops of essential oil in approximately 4 ounces of dried milk powder, whole milk, or Epson salts. Add mixture to bathtub while filling with warm water. Soak in bath for 10 to 20 minutes. Because essential oils are not water-soluble, this mixture allows for essential oils to disperse evenly in the bath.

Compress: A warm or cold compress may be used. Add 2 to 6 drops of essential oil to a basin of water and stir. Place cloth or gauze in basin and soak. Wring out the cloth or gauze and apply directly on the affected area. Repeat as needed.

Cosmetics Addition: When carrier oil is unavailable, essential oils may be added to fragrance and chemical-free lotions, such as shea butter, massage cream, or jojoba butter. Use 40 to 48 drops per 4 ounces of moisturizer. If skin is sensitive or if you plan to use on children, fewer drops of essential oil is recommended.

Direct Application: Essential oils can be directly applied to the skin using a dilution of 40 to 48 drops of essential oil in 4 ounces of carrier oil. One to 4 drops of some essential oils may be used safely undiluted on the skin. If skin is sensitive or if you plan to use on children, fewer drops of essential oil are recommended. Apply about 1/2 ounce of oil for each application.

Foot Bath: Add 2 to 6 drops of essential oil to a basin of cool or warm water, and mix the water vigorously. Soak feet for 10 to 20 minutes.

Massage: Dilute the essential oils as follows:

For adults: Forty to 48 drops of essential oil in 4 ounces of carrier oil or fragrance and chemical-free lotion, depending on skin sensitivity. If skin is sensitive, fewer drops of essential oil are recommended. Apply about 1/2 ounce of oil for each application.

For children: Less than 2 years: 5 to 10 drops of essential oil in 4 ounces of carrier oil or lotion. Over age 2 years: 10 to 20 drops of essential oil in 4 ounces of carrier oil or lotion.

Oral (Taken by Mouth) Applications

Ingestion of essential oils is NOT recommended unless under the observation and care of a knowledgeable health professional of aromatherapy. Extreme precaution should be taken when ingesting essential oils and should be especially avoided in small children under the age of six.

Mouth Wash: Add 2 to 6 drops of essential oil to 4 ounces of water. Swish around mouth and spit out. Do not swallow.

Oral Mist: Add 2 to 6 drops of essential oil in 4 ounces of water into a mister bottle. If preferred, aloe vera gel may be added to the mist.

Buying and Storage

The essential oil bottle should state the plant species from which the oil is derived. Only use essential oils from a reputable supplier who provides information assuring the product is 100% pure essential oil by gas chromatography-mass spectrometry analysis. Pure essential oils are expensive to produce and therefore tend to be costly.

Although there are no expiration dates on essential oils, exposure to air, heat, and light may decrease their effectiveness. Store essential oils in colored (amber or blue) glass bottles with orifice reducer inserts and tight fitting lids in a cool, dark place. If the reducer insert is not available, use a pipette for precise measurement when dispensing an essential oil.

Choosing an Aromatherapy Remedy that is Right for You

Ideally, start with an essential oil that smells pleasant and an aromatherapy application that is both comfortable and convenient for you. If relief is not obtained with 2 to 3 applications, you can experiment with additional essential oils or applications or choose another therapy.

Cautions with Essential Oils

• Do not touch your eyes when handling essential oils. Always wash your hands well after use.

• Citrus essential oils may increase your sensitivity to the sun; avoid topical application of these oils prior to sun exposure.

• Be aware that essential oils are oil-based products and may cause staining of clothes, sheets, or any cloth-based item.

• Keep essential oils out of reach of children.

• In rare cases, essential oils may be associated with other specific side effects. For more specific information about side effects associated aromatherapy, you can find detailed information in the *People's Desk Reference for Essential Oils* (Appendix I).

• Avoid the following list of essential oils during pregnancy: Angelica, Basil, Calamus, Celery Seed, Cinnamon Bark, Citronella, Clary Sage, Eucalyptus, Fennel, Hyssop, Marjoram, Nutmeg, Palo Santo, Rosemary, Sage, Tansy Idaho, Tarragon, and Wintergreen.

Remember a drop of essential oil goes a long way.

Chinese Medicine and Acupressure

Chinese medicine is a complete medical system dating back more than 5,000 years. Chinese medicine is based on a unique understanding of health and disease, which uses a detailed and complex system of physiological and pathological processes. Chinese medicine is fundamentally established on the principles of yin and yang, the existence and flow of "qi" (*pronounced chee*) within the body, and the idea that the elements which occur in nature (wind, fire, cold, damp, dryness), can also occur in the body and impact physiological function. Yin and yang serve as a pair of opposites, each needing the other to exist in the same manner as we need night to understand day; cold to understand hot; stillness to understand movement. The foundation of Chinese medicine is to keep yin and yang in perfect balance.

Qi is an important diagnostic feature of Chinese medicine. Qi is a vital substance that provides the physiological basis for all bodily functions. The health of an individual's qi is impacted by lifestyle, which is affected by the air we breathe and the food and drink we consume. Qi flows through a complex meridian system reaching all areas of the body and can be accessed and manipulated through therapeutic points (acupoints). Each meridian is associated with a biological organ. There are 14 meridians and 361 different acupoints located on these meridians. Acupoints are named for the meridian on which they fall and are numbered sequentially. For example, the acupoint ST 36 is the 36th point on the Stomach meridian.

The development of disease is distinctly different according to Chinese medicine when compared to conventional medicine. According to Chinese medicine, a pathogen can invade the body from the outside (wind, heat, cold, dampness and dryness) as in the case of the common cold, which is a more similar approach to conventional medicine. However, disease can also develop by a disruption to the flow of qi and imbalances of yin and yang. Chinese medicine emphasizes balance in all aspects of life as a pathway to achieving health. This involves both moderation and self-cultivation. Disruption in balance can be caused by poor lifestyle habits (diet, little exercise, overwork, stress), extreme, long term or unresolved emotional disruption, or trauma/accidents.

Chinese medicine treatments include the use of acupuncture, herbs, tui na (massage), moxibustion (application of heat), diet and exercise (qi gong). The choice of meridians and points for a therapeutic indication can vary slightly depending on the philosophy of the Chinese medicine practitioner. Within Chinese medicine there are a number of different treatment philosophies. Practitioners can apply one philosophy or rely on a combination of philosophies to develop treatment principles. Some of the most common philosophies of Chinese medicine are Traditional Chinese Medicine (TCM), Five Element Acupuncture, Japanese or Korean Acupuncture, and Trigger Point Therapy. In this book we present acupoints that are based on TCM philosophy, and certain dietary strategies based on TCM diet therapy.

Acupuncture

Acupuncture is probably the most common TCM modality used in both Asia and the United States. It is the insertion of fine gauge needles into acupoints in order to access the meridians where qi flows throughout the body and to elicit a therapeutic result. **Acupuncture is not a self-help therapy.** You should only accept treatment from an experienced acupuncturist licensed in the state where you receive treatment. **Do not receive acupuncture from an unlicensed acupuncturist.** Acupuncturists can be identified by the initials following their name. These can vary by state, but typically a licensed acupuncturist will hold the title of LAc. Medical doctors, and in some states other health professionals, can also practice a simplified form of acupuncture; however, these programs do not provide education on all aspects of acupuncture theory and practice.

Acupressure

Acupressure is a self-help therapy that can be applied by the patient upon proper instruction. Although acupressure and acupuncture use the same points on the body, acupressure differs in that fingers are used to stimulate the acupoints on the surface of the skin. No penetration is necessary. Although acupressure can be very effective, acupuncture often has a more pronounced effect and may be indicated if conditions do not resolve with acupressure.

Applying acupressure

This book provides the reader with a series of acupoints to be used in a hospital or home setting. The most challenging aspect of using acupressure is identification of the acupoint. Appendix A includes illustrations of each acupoint listed in this book along with brief directions to identify each acupoint. If you do not obtain relief, add the secondary acupoints for an additional therapeutic effect.

Once you have located the area of the acupoint, use the thumb or forefinger and apply light to medium pressure. If it is difficult to identify the point, palpate around the area to find the point of tenderness or fullness. The right amount of pressure will depend on the acupoint and the sensitivity of the individual. If the pressure is uncomfortable, lighten the pressure. A minimum amount of pressure should be at least the weight of a medium size coin. Use your thumb to massage or press the area. Applying acupressure to the surrounding area of the acupoint will also have therapeutic value. In general, you can continue to apply pressure until the symptom is relieved, or you can hold it for a few minutes up to several times a day. It is best to have someone else do this for you, using both hands, and applying acupressure. This technique is illustrated below.

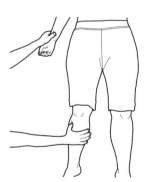

If you are using a specific acupoint repeatedly, indicating the acupoint with a fine tip pen or marker may be helpful for subsequent sessions.

Cautions with Acupressure

Acupressure should be avoided in areas that are inflamed, swollen, bruised, or burned. Acupressure should not be applied directly on open wounds or directly into tumor masses. Acupressure points that stimulate labor and delivery points should be avoided in women who are pregnant. If you are pregnant, avoid GB 21, LI 4, Liv 3, SP 6, UB 60, UB 67.

Herbal Teas

Herbal teas, often referred to as medicinal teas, are brewed from flowers, leafy parts of plants (except *Camellia sinensis*), roots, barks, seeds, twigs, or berries, rather than the actual tea plant leaves. Some practitioners prefer administration of herbal teas over capsulated herbs for greater exposure to all therapeutic aspects of the plant. In this book we refer to herbal teas made from all plant and fruit parts.

The manufacture of bagged teas for mass consumption was invented in the early 1900's to minimize the mess associated with the use of loose tea. Although preparation of tea using bags is still a very good way of making tea, prepackaged herbal tea bags sold at the supermarket generally crush all parts of the plant into pieces, which may dilute the tea's therapeutic benefit. Preparation of tea using herbs purchased in bulk is less subject to this complication. Although many of the more commonly prescribed herbal teas such as chamomile, peppermint, and ginger are available pre-packaged in most local supermarkets, we recommend purchasing bulk herbs and preparing the tea as described below.

Because teas can be brewed from various parts of an herbal plant, a few different brewing techniques are described. The infusion method is a simple technique to make tea using flowers and the leafy part of plants. The decoction method is a more labor-intensive method of making tea and is the recommended technique when making teas from roots, barks, seeds, twigs, and berries.

Items Needed to Make an Infusion

- Kettle
- Glass, glazed earthenware, or porcelain teapot
- Strainer or tea bag
- Teacup
- Fresh or dried loose tea

How to Make an Infusion

1. Break apart the herbs with a mortar and pestle, back of a spoon, or with your fingers.
2. Fill a tea kettle with fresh, cold water and set it on the stove, turning the burner to high.
3. Measure the amount of loose tea needed. Doses of the herbs for management of each side effect are indicated in the corresponding chapter.
4. Spoon the loose tea parts directly into the teapot, inset basket, or strainer. If using a homemade tea bag, spoon the loose tea parts inside the bag and drop into the teapot.
5. When the water just reaches a boil, pour the water into the teapot, steeping the tea as directed within each chapter.
6. Once steeping is complete, remove inset basket, strainer, or tea bag. If using loose tea, strain the tea over the tea cup and empty additional tea into teapot.

Items Needed to Make a Decoction

- Saucepan
- Strainer
- Teacup and/or pitcher
- Fresh or dried loose tea

How to Make a Decoction

1. Chop or cut roots, bark, or twigs into small pieces. Bruise berries and seeds with a mortar and pestle, back of a spoon, or with your fingers.
2. Place the herb in a saucepan and add cold water.
3. Set the saucepan on the stove, turning the burner to high.
4. Bring to a gentle boil, reduce heat, and simmer for 10 minutes to 1 hour or until the volume has been reduced by one-third.
5. Strain the tea over the tea cup and/or pitcher.

Drink tea hot or cold. Teas may be prepared one to two days in advance. Store the herbal tea at room temperature and away from direct sunlight. After two days, prepare a fresh tea. Do not store at room temperature for more than two days.

Homeopathy

Homeopathy, also known as homeopathic medicine, is a whole medical system that was developed by the German doctor Samuel Christian Hahnemann in the late 18th century. Homeopathic remedies are based on natural substances derived from plants, animals, and minerals and prepared in a series of dilutions. Homeopathy was developed using the "principle of similars" and the concept of "potentization." The "principle of similars" states that any sign or symptom elicited from a plant or mineral will be an antidote for diseases that present with similar signs or symptoms. For example, the plant poison ivy produces redness, itching and swelling. Dilutions of that same plant would be used to treat illnesses that produce similar symptoms. Another underlying principle of homeopathy is that a remedy is more effective when the vital essence of the substance is extracted by systematically diluting a substance and vigorously shaking the remedy between dilutions.

Homeopathic remedies are individualized and based on the concept of holism and the totality of symptoms. According to traditional homeopathy, a homeopath makes a diagnosis by evaluating all aspects of the individual (physical symptoms, emotions, mental states, lifestyle and nutrition) and not just symptoms of the disease. Therefore, homeopaths may prescribe different remedies for people experiencing the same symptom. However, some homeopaths practice a more uniform approach in making a diagnosis, with the underlying tenets of homeopathic medicine driving more generalized recommendations that are applicable for everyone, similar to a conventional approach to the treatment of a sign or symptom.

Regulations for homeopathy vary by country. In 1938, a law was passed by Congress requiring homeopathic remedies to be regulated by the U.S. Food and Drug Administration (FDA) as over-the-counter drugs, which allows their purchase without a doctor's prescription. Since 1988, the FDA has required all homeopathic remedies to list their ingredients, dilutions and indications and instructions for safe use.

Homeopathic remedies are available in liquid, pellet, tablet or topical forms. Remedies are sold at various strengths (6x, 12x, 30x or 24c, 100c). A higher number indicates a more dilute yet "potent" remedy. In practice, a stronger dose does not necessarily equate to greater efficacy for the condition being treated. Remedies may be recommended to be taken repetitively within a short time-frame; for example, one or two pellets every 15 minutes or daily.

For chronic conditions, a lower potency is often prescribed for a longer period of time. For more acute conditions (for example: a throbbing headache), a stronger dilution will be prescribed many times within a shorter time frame.

Choosing the Homeopathic Remedy that is Right for You

There are two approaches in choosing a homeopathic remedy. Traditionally, homeopaths evaluate a totality of symptoms in prescribing the appropriate remedy. However, some homeopaths prescribe an antidote much in the same way a practitioner would use a nutrition or herbal supplement. In this book, we most often provide both approaches. Homeopathic remedies that are most frequently prescribed by homeopathic practitioners are in bold. For each remedy, we also provide additional signs and symptoms that may make a specific remedy more appropriate for the side effect you are experiencing. Start with the remedy in bold. You can also choose the remedy that best describes the symptom you are experiencing. If relief is not obtained, choose a different complementary therapy.

If you experience improvement in your symptoms, discontinue the remedy. Resume remedy if symptom recurs. In general, if you are experiencing severe and acute symptoms, frequent repetition (dose every 15 to 30 minutes for a specified period of time) is an important treatment principal. For chronic symptoms, fewer repetitions (dose once or twice per day) are recommended. Depending on the potency and condition, a remedy is typically not administered for longer than 7 to 14 days. Depending on the side effect, relief should be experienced within 24–48 hours for acute conditions and up to 7 to 14 days for persistent or chronic conditions. If no relief is experienced after seven days, select another homeopathic remedy that best describes your symptoms or choose another therapy for managing the side effect. Consultation with a professional homeopath may also be considered. Dosing for each side effect is provided in the corresponding chapter.

Cautions with Homeopathy

Use of any supplement, including homeopathic remedies, could potentially interfere with the efficacy of cancer therapy. Please refer to the section entitled Supplements in this chapter for more information regarding the risks associated with homeopathic remedies. Consider consulting with an expert in the field of homeopathy. In the United States, there is no uniform consensus for the qualifications necessary for the practice of homeopathy, and credentialing for homeopaths varies by state. Homeopathic schools may be a resource for identifying qualified practitioners in your area. Resources to identify homeopathic schools are available in Appendix I.

Massage

Massage therapy is one of the most popular complementary medicine therapies used in cancer care. Most of the great ancient cultures of the world have recorded the use of massage or rubbing techniques; Egyptians, Persians, and Japanese historical writings and artifacts often refer to the practice. Chinese pediatric massage dates back to the Sui/Tang dynasty (A.D. 581–907), and Hippocrates described massage as "medicine being the art of rubbing." The gladiators were known to receive massage prior to their performances to enhance blood flow and mental awareness.

Massage can provide physical, emotional and mental relaxation for not only the patient, but for his or her family members and other caregivers. Massage relieves muscle tension and reduces pain, which may then enhance feelings of deep relaxation and well-being. According to massage theory, physical and emotional pain can reduce the circulation of blood and nervous system communication in the body. By stimulating blood flow and release of endorphins (the body's own natural painkillers), immediate relaxation is experienced. Massage can help in the management of both acute (very sensitive, severe, of short duration) and chronic conditions (long lasting, always present, long term). Massage may be especially helpful with recovery from surgery due to local trauma of the soft tissue.

Many forms of massage therapy are practiced in the United States; at least 150 methods from various regions around the world may be employed. The most popular forms of massage are Swedish, Deep Tissue, Medical Massage, Sports Massage, Shiatsu, Tui Na, Reflexology, and Manual Lymphatic Drainage. These styles are distinguished by the underlying theory guiding the depth and form of stroke. This book focuses on Swedish massage, a simple system of hands-on strokes one can use with or without oil or moisturizer.

We present three basic strokes of Swedish massage in this book. In each chapter, we recommend specific muscles or body areas to be massaged to help manage each side effect. Before administering self-massage or massage to another person, make sure the person is in a comfortable position. If the person is uncomfortable lying flat, try to administer massage with the person lying on the side or sitting upright.

Effleurage (Figure 1)

This is a wide hand stroke usually accompanied with oil or moisturizer, such as sliding down the whole back or sliding up the leg. Effleurage should be done first, and generally with a lighter touch than the two other strokes. The purpose of effleurage is to warm up the area by getting the circulation moving. It also helps initiate the relaxation process.

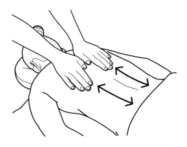

Figure 1.

Pettrisage (Figure 2)

This is a more specific hand stroke and is the most commonly used stroke. The pressure is a little deeper than effleurage, thereby penetrating into the connective tissue and muscles. A smaller area of the body, specific to a muscle group, is covered such as the muscles around the shoulder area.

Pettrisage is used to loosen up an area of tight muscles or pain. It may also help with an internal problem. For instance, in the case of shortness of breath, symptoms may improve with massage over the chest. Constipation may be relieved by massage over the

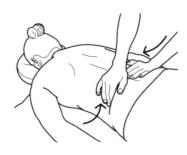

Figure 2.

belly. Since the massage technique is applied with a deeper pressure, it can be felt more than the effleurage technique.

Friction (Figure 3)

This is the most specific of the three techniques. Friction should be applied with medium to deep pressure. A very small area, commonly called a "knot," the most sensitive and tender part of the muscle, is treated. Use the thumb or another finger to press on the knot. The thumb or finger then moves across it with small, specific, deep strokes, similar to strumming a guitar string. The thumb or finger may also follow the direction of the muscle to potentially loosen the muscle fibers in a process referred to as muscle stripping. You can also simply press down on the "knot" and hold for about 10 seconds. Release, repeat the sequence two or three times for each identified "knot." This requires no movement other than pressure.

If further education on massage techniques is desired, consult with a licensed massage therapist. In most states, practitioners must be licensed to practice massage therapy (massage qualifications are denoted as LMT, licensed massage therapist). Guidance on finding a licensed practitioner in your area can be found in Appendix I.

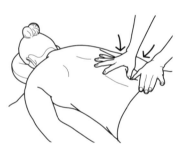

Figure 3.

Cautions with Massage

Special care should be taken before massaging yourself or a family member. Avoid massaging on the following areas:

- Directly over any tumor mass.
- Areas that are red, inflamed, or burned from radiation therapy
- Any open wounds, bruises, or over any irritated skin.
- Scars less than 2 to 4 weeks old. Massage should only be applied after the acute phase of recovery (2 to 4 weeks).

- Acute deep venous thrombosis. For blood clots located on the lower body, avoid massaging the lower body. Massage only the upper limbs, neck, shoulder, back, and chest. For blood clots located on upper body, massage only the chest and back. Do not massage any of the four limbs.

If you have neuropathy or numbness, caution should be taken to avoid deep pressure because you may not be able to sense uncomfortable pressure that may be associated with massage. Special caution must be taken among individuals who are experiencing lymphedema or at risk for developing lymphedema. Certain forms of massage therapy such as rolfing, deep tissue massage, shiatsu, and tui na are not safe for individuals with lymphedema or at risk for developing lymphedema. **Manual lymphatic drainage is the only accepted form of massage therapy for prevention and treatment of lymphedema.** Other forms of massage therapy may be used such as, reflexology, and Swedish massage; however, these forms must be administered by a licensed massage therapist and under the supervision of your medical oncologist. Special caution should be taken if you had abdominal surgery. Do not massage on the affected area until consulting with your doctor. If you are pregnant, no massage should be administered on the lower belly and back in the 1st trimester. In the 2nd and 3rd trimester, avoid massage on the belly.

Nutrition

Nutrition is the study and science of how nutrients found in food affect biological actions within the body. The nutrients from food can be from animal or plant sources, and are needed to provide energy, sustain growth and development, and promote daily biological functions. We need more than 40 required nutrients for our bodies to function; these mandatory nutrients include carbohydrates, protein, fat, and many vitamins and minerals such as calcium, folate, vitamin C and vitamin D. The Dietary Reference Intakes (DRI) are nutrient reference values established by experts in the Institute of Medicine to serve as a guide for minimum nutrient intake for healthy individuals. The DRIs are not designed to meet the nutrient needs of individuals with any medical condition. The DRIs serves as a guide for monitoring daily intakes of vitamins and minerals, and are used as a reference when planning and evaluating diets. Other variables considered when evaluating dietary plans are medical conditions, ethnic background, socioeconomic status, cultural traditions, life stage, and psychological status.

Nutrition plays an important role over the spectrum of cancer care. Scientists estimate that nearly 70% of cancers may be prevented with good nutrition and a healthy lifestyle, and have found that during cancer therapy, poor nutrition status (a decrease of >5% of normal body weight and/or decreased muscle or protein stores) can make the side effects associated with cancer therapy much worse. Eating a diet that at least meets the recommended DRI for your age will improve energy levels and overall quality of life during cancer treatment. After therapy, healthy dietary habits, as part of a healthy lifestyle, can decrease the risk of the development of a late effect of cancer treatment or prevent recurrence.

Nutrition is the only therapy presented in this book that is an integral component of both conventional and many complementary treatments. Therefore, deciphering "conventional" versus "complementary" nutrition can be complicated. Historically, nutrition has been used as a treatment for a variety of illnesses. In ancient times the Greeks referred to food as a form of medicine. In TCM, diet changes are frequently the back bone of the treatment plans. Today many nutrition interventions are essential components of disease management; some examples include high fiber diets for diabetes, low fat diets for prevention of heart disease, and intravenous nutrition for the treatment of moderate to severe malnutrition.

Conventional nutrition therapy consists of education and advanced intervention. Nutrition education provides patients information on foods and nutrients; whereas, advanced nutrition interventions include the use of nutrition formulas, tube feeding or feeding through an intravenous route. There is a great deal of information available on nutrition during and after cancer therapy including several online resources. The National Cancer Institute (http://www.cancer.gov/cancertopics/pdq/supportivecare/nutrition/patient) and American Institute for Cancer Research (www.aicr.org) provide patient information on the role of nutrition during and after cancer therapy. These websites also provide information on dietary guidance to help manage symptoms associated with cancer therapy.

A nutritionist or dietician can help guide you on the basics of nutrition therapy during and after treatment for cancer. Nutritionists may hold a variety of degrees. Most commonly, nutrition practitioners are MD (Medical Doctor), RD (Registered Dietician), ND (Doctor of Naturopathic Medicine), or LAc (Licensed Acupuncturist). Variations in the nutrition recommendations will reflect the training and clinical theory of the practitioner. Typically a LAc will practice diet therapy from a TCM approach; whereas most MDs and RDs will exercise a more conventional approach. A member of your medical team may be able to provide you with a list of recommended practitioners in nutrition therapy. Prior to arranging an appointment, investigate whether the practitioner is experienced and knowledgeable in working with patients undergoing cancer therapy, and is willing to communicate with your conventional medical team. Choose a practitioner that makes you comfortable, that you understand, and with whom you agree on the framework of the recommendations. This will be important in successfully adopting any new dietary plan.

This book provides the reader with an overview of foods that may help in managing cancer treatment related symptoms. The recommendations are not suggested to treat cancer. The nutrition recommendations can be used in conjunction with conventional care recommendations and emphasize foods that are minimally processed and prepared and consumed in a way that confers the most nutrient benefit. Some of the foods included in this book have been used historically to manage the indicated sign or symptom. Others are driven from clinical research or practice. Choose a few recommendations that are most comfortable and familiar to you so that they will require the least amount of effort on your part. If you are not experiencing relief, you might consider some of the additional suggestions. Many of the foods are available at your local supermarket, market, or health food store. Be open, patient, and allow yourself to experiment with new flavors and textures. You might be surprised by what you discover!

A Brief Word About Advanced Forms of Nutrition Intervention

Advanced nutrition intervention is often required during cancer therapy. Examples of advanced forms of nutrition intervention are the use of appetite stimulants (Cyproheptadine (Periactin®), Dronabinal (Marinol®), megestrol acetate (Megace®), dexamethasone (Decadron)), enteral feeding (delivering food through a tube into the stomach), or intravenous nutrition (administration of nutrients through an intravenous catheter). Each of these interventions requires the oversight and management by your doctor and medical team. Some complementary medicine providers promote the use of intravenous forms of nutrition. It is important that you speak with your doctor before engaging in these practices.

Complementary/Alternative Diets

Many complementary/alternative diets are promoted as a treatment for cancer, support during cancer therapy, or cancer prevention. Examples of complementary/alternative diets are: The Raw Foods Diet, Macrobiotics, Suzanne Somers Diet, or Gonzalez Regimen. Typically, complementary/alternative diets are part of a therapeutic regimen that can include the use of dietary supplements (herbal and/or nutrition), enemas, juicing, herbal teas, or detoxification. These diets may promote organic, locally grown foods, and may also emphasize lifestyle modifications such as mind/body exercises.

Few clinical trials have investigated the efficacy or safety of most complementary/alternative dietary regimens. If you are seeking to cure your cancer with nutrition, speak with your doctor first. **There is no evidence that any dietary regimen treats cancer.** If you are interested in these dietary regimens in addition to your current diet, consult with a dietician or nutritionist. Because deficiencies in either macronutrients or micronutrients can occur when following a strict diet, a modification may be necessary. A consultation will ensure that you will be able to meet your nutrient requirements.

Some complementary/alternative diets include enemas as part of a therapeutic regimen. Enemas can be dangerous without medical oversight especially in patients with low platelet counts or neutropenia (low white blood cell counts). Consult with your doctor before choosing to use any type of enema.

Reflexology

Reflexology is a science and art of reflex points on the feet, hands and ears. These points correspond to every organ, gland, muscle and bone in the body. Reflexology dates as far back as 2330 BC. Hieroglyphics were found in an Egyptian tomb depicting doctors of the time giving reflexology to the hands and feet of pharaohs. From there reflexology traveled to India, China, and Japan. Franciscan missionaries in the Far East brought this technique to Europe, and at the turn of the 20th century it was brought to America.

Central to reflexology therapy is the notion that stimulation of the reflex points enhances circulation and balances the nervous system. According to the theory of reflexology, the body is divided into ten vertical lines or zones (Appendix C). Each zone is considered an invisible "highway" that allows energy to flow freely throughout the body. There are ten zones that begin and end on either the fingers or toes. Each zone contains reflex points that are located on the hands or feet, and it is through these points that the energy in the zone can be accessed and manipulated. Reflex points correspond to every organ, gland, muscle, or bone in the body. Disharmony can cause a block in a zone, which can present as symptoms of pain or dysfunction, anxiety, stress, fatigue or other medical ailments. When the reflex point is accessed by using a pressure technique with the thumb or finger, the associated ailment is treated. The pressure can be light or deep. The pressure is more for comfort rather than for therapeutic effectiveness.

There is no national board certification standard for reflexology in the United States. Laws governing reflexologists vary by state. In some states, reflexology falls under the domain of massage therapy. If seeking a qualified practitioner explore the American Reflexology Certification Board Website (ARCB) for a list of nationally certified practitioners (Appendix I).

Application of Reflexology

Reflexology can be performed in a chair, bed, or lying on the floor. It is best if the person is lying down so he or she can relax; however, reflexology can be applied when the person is sitting or standing, if necessary. The primary techniques used are the finger walking technique, hooking technique, rotation on a point, and thumb walking. In general, the thumb technique is more appropriate for fleshier areas, the finger technique is best suited for small or bony areas, and the hooking and rotation on a point techniques are used for reflex areas that are found deep in the muscle tissue. For example, use the thumb technique for the palmar (the palm of the hand) and plantar (bottom of the foot) surfaces and the finger technique for the dorsal (top) sides of the hands and feet. For ease of administration, it is helpful to hold the foot or hand with one of your hands while applying pressure to a specific point with the other. Reflexology is generally preferred over massage for infants, young children, and weak adults, or if the local area of discomfort cannot be touched directly on the body.

The theory of reflexology states that the right hand and foot correspond to the right side of the body, and the left hand and foot correspond to the left side of the body. If an organ, muscle or gland is found on both sides of the body, it will be reflected in both the hands and feet. However, if there is only a one-sided organ, such as the spleen, the reflex will only be found on one hand or foot. If an organ or gland is found in the center of the body, such as the brain or spine, then half of the reflex will be on one hand or foot while the other half will be on the other hand or foot. Refer to reflexology illustrations for specification. Below is a brief description of the four primary reflexology techniques:

Finger walking (Figure 4)

Finger walking technique is the same as thumb walking technique except the pointer finger is used for bony areas of the hands and feet while the thumb is used for fleshier areas. Both techniques look like an inchworm.

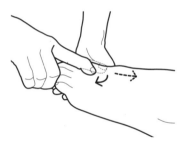

Figure 4.

Hooking technique (Figure 5)

This is for accessing a point on the deepest level. Place your thumb on the point and press directly onto the point while supporting the foot or hand with your other hand. After

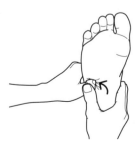

Figure 5.

placing your thumb on the point, hook in with your thumb either to the right or left, depending on which foot or hand you are working with. This technique is used on the pineal, pituitary, thymus, hypothalamus and ilocecal valve reflexes only.

Rotation on a point (Figure 6)

Use rotation on a point when your finger strength cannot be sustained with thumb walking or finger walking or if you simply want deeper pressure. This is a technique where you find a particular point and place your thumb on it. Point descriptions are found within each chapter. With the other hand, you rotate the whole foot or hand on top of the point. You can rotate the foot in a clockwise or counter clockwise direction, whatever is easier for you.

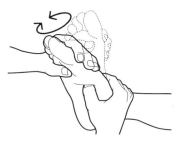

Figure 6.

Thumb walking (Figure 7)

Thumb walking looks like you are using your thumb as an inchworm across an area on the foot or hand. Press the side or pad of your thumb on a specific area, open the joint, close the joint, open the joint, close the joint. This looks like you are inching your way across or up the foot or hand. The purpose of thumb walking is to move along different areas of the foot without taking off pressure for optimal effect.

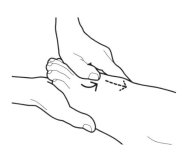

Figure 7.

The following key indicates which technique is used for a point or area on the foot or hand and will be indicated in each section of the chapter:

F = finger walking technique
H = hooking technique
R = rotation on a point
T = thumb walking technique

Cautions of Reflexology

The same cautions for massage are applied to reflexology. Refer to the massage section in this chapter.

Supplements (Nutrition, Herbal)

Dietary supplements are products that can be nutrient-based (nutrition supplements) or plant-based (herbal supplements). Nutrition supplements may contain vitamins, minerals, amino acids, or enzymes whereas herbal supplements are products containing herbs (also referred to as botanicals) either alone or in mixtures (nccam.nih.gov). The term "herb" when used medically refers to any part of the plant used for therapeutic purposes. Nutrition supplements are designed to supplement the diet with nutrients, not serve as a replacement for a healthy diet. Dietary supplements are available in capsule, tablet, extract, powder, tea, cream or ointment form. How they are administered is often practitioner-dependent; for example, practitioners of TCM advocate the use of teas and extracts whereas many Western practitioners promote the use of capsules or tablets.

Risks Associated with Dietary Supplements

Contamination of dietary supplements

In the United States, dietary supplements are regulated as food products and not as medications, as long as there are no specific claims for action against a specific disease. For example, a dietary supplement may be marketed as "supporting immune function" but cannot be marketed for "curing breast cancer" without going through rigorous scientific evaluation to support that claim.

The benefit of this regulation for the consumer and supplier is that dietary supplements are more readily available since manufacturers do not have to follow the long and rigorous evaluation process that is required for new drugs. However, the downside of this limited regulation is that dietary supplements are not required to adhere to the Good Manufacturing Practices (GMP) that regulated medications are required by law to follow. Unfortunately this means that some dietary supplements may be contaminated with other medications (for example, some Chinese herbs have been found to be contaminated with prescription medications) or may not contain the amount of herb or nutrient indicated on the label (for example, a product may state on the label it contains 100 mg of a nutrient, but the product only contains 50 mg). Dietary supplements may be contaminated with heavy metals such as lead, which can be especially problematic for young children whose brains are still developing. Some herbs have also been found to contain fungi or bacteria, a potential concern for patients undergoing treatment for cancer because a decreased immune system is a side effect of many cancer therapies.

Fortunately some dietary supplement manufacturers voluntarily adhere to GMP practices and/or have been tested by outside agencies such as Consumer Labs® which performs independent testing on dietary supplements focusing on ingredients, dosage, and contamination. Choosing dietary supplements that adhere to these standards will decrease but not completely avoid the risks of contamination and mislabeling.

Interactions with cancer therapy

Using dietary supplements during active treatment for cancer is controversial. Your doctor may be concerned about combining dietary supplements with conventional therapy because for most dietary supplements, the safety of this approach is not known. Although some dietary supplements may help make cancer therapy more effective, some supplements may decrease the effectiveness of the cancer therapy. Dietary supplements may also increase the side effects of cancer treatment. Unfortunately, there is not much information from scientific studies to guide decisions about using dietary supplements during cancer therapy.

It is very important to speak with your doctor about your interest in taking dietary supplements during cancer therapy [*Refer to Chapter 2: Communicating with your doctor and complementary medicine provider*]. A thorough discussion of the risks and benefits of combining dietary supplements with cancer care should be held with your doctor. The risks of a dietary supplement interacting with cancer therapy are greater if the dietary supplement is used during the entire conventional treatment period, if multiple dietary supplements are taken at the same time, or if intravenous or high doses of any dietary supplement are administered. In this book, the most commonly used supplements for a specific indication are in bold. Some of the supplements highlighted in bold have research supporting their safety and/or efficacy.

If you and your doctor decide to use dietary supplements during therapy, there are some steps you can take to reduce the risk of an interaction.

• Dietary supplements with a DRI. Strive to meet the recommendations for dietary supplements with a DRI. Tables of DRI values may be found on the Institute of Medicine website at http://www.iom.edu/CMS/54133/54377.aspx.
• Dietary supplements with no DRI. In these cases, you can work with your doctor, complementary therapy provider or pharmacist to work out a schedule for taking your

dietary supplements, based on the clearance (often referred to as "half lives") of the chemotherapy agents and the dietary supplements. In such circumstances, work with your doctor and complementary medicine provider to determine the safest dose, ideally based on evidence from clinical trials.

• Dietary supplements with scientific studies supporting efficacy for a specific sign or symptom. Work with your doctor and complementary provider and determine a dose based on the clinical study. Depending on your age and clinical condition, this may require modification.

Most recommendations for dietary supplements are based on anecdotal or historical practice. In this setting your doctor and complementary therapy provider should closely monitor for warning signs of an adverse interaction. This may include an increased or decreased frequency or severity of the expected side effects associated with cancer therapy or a delay in expected time to remission from the cancer.

Visual Imagery

Visual imagery refers to the practice of imagining or creating an image in your mind and holding that image for a specific effect. Visual imagery is a mind-body medicine discipline that can be readily integrated into conventional care. Visual imagery bridges the brain, mind, and body, directly promoting relaxation and affecting health. The theory behind visual imagery is that energy follows thought. If you think of something and hold that thought, it can manifest physically in your body or your life. By creating a new situation in your body with your mind, you replace the old one. If you find your thoughts wandering, re-create the vision and pick up where you left off or start again.

The healing concept that the mind is important in the treatment of emotional and physical illness has historically been used for over 2,000 years in TCM and in Indian Ayurvedic medicine. Hippocrates (400 B.C.), the father of modern conventional medicine also held that treatment for an illness could only occur by taking into account mental and emotional attitudes and environmental influences.

Visual imagery is not affiliated with any religion or spiritual practice and is a generally safe therapy for all ages. Visualizations may need to be modified for toddlers or young children. In this book, specific visual imageries have been developed for most of the side effects presented. A CD including all guided visualizations may also be purchased (*Integrative Strategies for Cancer Patients: A Companion of Guided Visual Imageries*, Eds: Elena J Ladas, Kara M Kelly).

In order to create an environment that is comfortable for you to practice visual imagery, find a quiet place where you will not be interrupted. Turn off your phone, radio or TV. Visual imagery can be done any time of the day or night. However, some time periods are better than others. For instance if you find you cannot sleep, try the visualization at the end of the day before bedtime. If you find you are tired and want to be energized, do the visualization in the morning or afternoon so you can experience the benefits. Some prefer to do the same visualization at the same time each day to set up a rhythm.

Each visual imagery exercise presented in this book takes at least 10 minutes and can go up to a half hour or longer if you prefer. If you find you cannot hold a thought for very long or you find yourself falling asleep or you cannot concentrate at all, do not worry. Keep practicing. Keep trying. Eventually you will get used to the imagery, and it will become easier. The more often you do it, the stronger you become and the more effective it can be. It may be helpful to combine visual imagery with aromatherapy to create a more peaceful and calming space.

Since visualizations are most often done with your eyes closed, we recommend that you review the provided text of the imagery several times in order to practice the steps from memory. You can also have someone slowly read and guide you through the visualization or you could record yourself reading it and play the visual imagery back to yourself. Guided audios of the visualizations in this book can also be purchased (Appendix I).

Additional resources on visual imagery may be found in Appendix I.

Yoga

Yoga is a physical and mental form of exercise that originated in India thousands of years ago. The word yoga is derived from the Sanskrit root "yuj" meaning to bind, or join together. Yoga combines both physical movement and breathing exercises to attain spiritual enlightenment, promote concentration, and achieve health and relaxation. Yoga aims to connect the movement of the body and the fluctuations of the mind to the rhythm of the breath. Yoga is useful in managing a variety of physical and mental health conditions, including asthma, hypertension, insomnia, stress, pain, anxiety, and depression. Yoga has a long history in improving overall quality of life and physical fitness, including cardiovascular fitness, flexibility, and strength.

There are many different forms of yoga practice; however, the philosophy of yoga is universal. This book focuses on Hatha yoga, the most commonly practiced form of yoga in the United States. Hatha yoga emphasizes yoga postures (asanas) and breathing exercises (pranayama) to achieve health and spirituality. There are many different disciplines of Hatha yoga including Iyengar yoga, Ashtanga yoga, Vinyasa (power yoga), Kundalini yoga, Bikram yoga (hot yoga) and Restorative yoga (supportive yoga). Each of these disciplines emphasizes a slightly different approach to the practice of Hatha yoga. For example, Iyengar yoga emphasizes alignment and precision in the asanas, Kundalini emphasizes breathwork and spirituality, and Restorative yoga emphasizes using props, bolsters, blocks and blankets to sustain a posture for a long time with ease and comfort. Restorative yoga helps facilitate deepening your breath, which in turn, nourishes and rests your body.

When yoga is indicated in the management of a specific side effect, a complete sequence of breathing exercises and yoga postures, also known as a vinyasa, are listed in the order to be practiced. Begin with the first yoga posture, and as you become comfortable, add additional yoga postures until you are able to perform the complete vinyasa. A comprehensive guide to the breathing exercises and yoga postures can be found in Appendix D. Step-by-step instructions as well as the level of difficulty, modifications and props, and cautions are provided for each breathing exercise and yoga posture. The level of difficulty is designated as beginner, intermediate, or advanced. If you have never practiced yoga, start with beginner breathing exercises and yoga postures and advance to more challenging poses as you become more comfortable and confident. For those with functional limitations or who would like their yoga practice to be more restorative, modifications and props are suggested to aid in completing a yoga pose.

Breathing Exercises (Pranayama)
Yoga breathing exercises emphasize the regulation of the breath in an effort to control the mind and attain mental clarity. What our brain perceives, our breath mirrors and our body experiences. Just as the mind influences the breath and body, so can the breath influence the mind and body. Controlling the power and rate of the breath is a technique called Pranayama. Breathing exercises covered in this book include Ujjayi breath, Kapalbhati, and Alternative nostril breathing. Breathing exercises should be practiced before yoga postures and are generally practiced while in a sitting position.

Yoga Postures (Asanas)
There are hundreds of yoga postures, each with many variations. Yoga postures stretch and align the body, strengthen bones, improve circulation, and promote balance and flexibility. Different yoga postures and variations in sequencing yoga postures offer unique benefits. In each chapter, we provide a suggested sequence of yoga postures for managing the specific condition. If you are unable to do the entire sequence, choose the postures you are able to do and follow the suggested order. The first time you do the vinyasa, stay in each posture for only a minimum number of breaths (about 1 to 5 breaths). Once you feel more comfortable, you can extend the length of your practice and stay in the postures for longer periods of time.

Yoga postures covered in this book can be categorized into seated postures, standing postures, balancing postures, twisting postures, restorative postures, backbends and inversions. Some postures fall into more than one category. Below is a brief description of each of the categories of yoga postures, and of the benefits of sun salutation, a preparatory sequence of yoga postures and positions.

Seated postures

These postures are the lowest level of difficulty and can accommodate any level of strength and flexibility. These postures develop elasticity to the knees, ankles and groin muscles and increase circulation of blood to the body. In seated postures the body is in position to achieve higher levels of relaxation because of ease of comfort of these postures.

Seated postures include: straight leg seated spinal twist, cobbler's pose, seated forward bend, child's pose

Standing postures

These postures are of varying levels of difficulty. These postures improve balance, strength and flexibility and will leave you feeling strong and grounded.

Standing postures include: mountain pose, prayer twist, tree pose, triangle pose, downward facing dog pose, chair pose, dancer's pose, standing forward bend, standing head to knee pose, revolving side angle pose, twisting triangle pose.

Balancing postures

These postures require varying levels of experience with yoga. These postures increase the capability of memory as well as improve concentration. They also achieve flexibility, strength, endurance, calmness, and mental clarity. Balancing yoga postures also help ease tension by transferring your focus to the present moment in order to perform the posture.

Balancing postures include: dancer's pose, standing head to knee pose, triangle pose, revolving side angle pose, twisting triangle pose, prayer twist, tree pose, chair pose.

Twisting postures

These postures require varying levels of experience with yoga. Twisting postures stretch the spine, shoulders, and hips and are a great way to relieve back and neck strain. These postures also massage the abdominal muscles, improve digestion, and relieve stress.

Twisting postures include: prayer twist, straight leg seated spinal twist, supine twist, twisting triangle pose, revolving side angle pose.

Back bends

These postures are recommended for intermediate and advanced levels. Back bends help energize, refresh and invigorate the body. Stretching the neck, stomach, and spine, back bends open the chest and encourage deep breathing. Back bends promote circulation to the heart and lungs and stimulate the nervous system, metabolism, and the lymphatic system.

Backbends include: bow pose, cobra pose, bridge pose, wheel pose, camel pose, dancer's pose, fish pose.

Inversions

These postures require *varying levels* of experience with yoga. Inversions are yoga postures that place the feet above the head. These postures are extremely useful in helping eliminate toxins from the body. It is believed that many impurities are stored in the lower belly, so by placing the feet above the head, the impurities are forced to move and make their way out of the body. These postures also help circulation and are great for strength and balance.

Inversions include: shoulderstand, headstand, legs up relaxation pose, plough pose.

Restorative postures

These postures are highly recommended for beginners, and patients who are in highly intensive phases of therapy in their treatment. Restorative postures focus on relaxing the body and mind. These postures help create equilibrium in the body either through normalizing heart rate and/or blood pressure, stimulating the immune system, or harmonizing the endocrine system. Almost any yoga posture can be made into a restorative posture by adding the right amount of supportive props. Supportive props are indicated for most yoga postures in Appendix D.

Classic restorative postures include: relaxation pose, legs up relaxation pose, supine knee squeeze, child's pose.

Sun salutation (Surya Namaskar)

The sun salutation is one of the most commonly practiced yoga posture sequences. The Sun Salutation synchronizes the breath through a dynamic sequence of yoga postures. Sun Salutation is generally used as a warm-up to a yoga posture session and is energizing, strengthening, and toning.

Sun Salutation yoga postures include: mountain pose, standing forward bend, downward facing dog pose, cobra pose.

Before You Begin

Choose the right ambience and attire before you begin your yoga practice. You will also need a yoga mat or a suitable alternative. You may find it helpful to wear comfortable, fitted clothing and to practice in a serene environment. Yoga is practiced barefoot; no special footgear is needed. It is preferable to practice yoga on an empty stomach, one hour after a light meal, or four hours after a heavy meal. Always breathe through your nose, not your mouth. As with any sport, interest, or hobby, the more you practice yoga, the greater the benefit.

Props

The use of yoga props will provide assistance in achieving the maximum benefit of poses during your yoga practice. Props are often not necessary if you are able to accomplish the pose. Props are indicated if you are experiencing difficulty in attaining the pose, physical limitations, including amputations or other post-surgical trauma, muscle atrophy, or lymphedema. Props may also be helpful if you are experiencing, fatigue, dizziness or difficulties with balance or coordination. The props presented in this book include: a straight back chair and wall (assist with balance), yoga straps (assist with stretch support), blocks or rolled up towels (assist with flexibility), and blankets (assist with restorative poses). Suggested props for specific yoga postures are provided in Appendix D.

Cautions with Yoga

You should not experience any pain when practicing breathing exercises and yoga postures. If you are not able to fully inhale and exhale in any posture, you are working too hard and should modify the posture so that you only feel slightly challenged. If you experience any sharp or stabbing sensations, numbness, shortness of breath, dizziness, or lightheadedness come out of the posture and rest in relaxation pose.

Specific cautions and contraindications for each breathing exercise and yoga posture are listed in Appendix D; however, there are some general cautions that you should take into consideration when beginning a yoga practice during cancer treatment.

• Avoid yoga postures that overly stretch the area around intravenous catheters (especially central venous catheters like Broviac or Hickman catheters, Mediports, Portacaths).

• Consult with your doctor following surgery. Advanced yoga postures should not be practiced immediately after surgery. Breathing exercises and restorative yoga postures that only require the use of body parts not part of the surgical procedure may be indicated.

• If you are experiencing respiratory issues, lightheadedness, or have low blood pressure avoid prolonged yoga standing and balancing poses.

• **Patients experiencing lymphedema or are at risk of developing lymphedema should discuss your yoga practice with your doctor.** You should gradually build the duration and intensity of your yoga practice. Take frequent rests between yoga postures by resting in relaxation pose which will allow for limb recovery. Wear your compression sleeve during your yoga practice.

• Avoid inversion poses if you are experiencing or are at risk for lymphedema or heart or lung complications.

Chapter 5
Cancer Associated Side Effects

Anxiety & Stress

What is Anxiety?

Adjusting to a diagnosis of cancer and the associated treatments can result in overwhelming stress that may lead to unpleasant feelings ranging from sadness to isolation. Too much stress commonly results in anxiety, the sudden or ongoing feeling of fear and uneasiness. Anxiety is a common emotional reaction experienced by patients with cancer. A person having anxiety may feel nauseous or restless, have a fast heartbeat, sweat, tremble, or experience poor concentration and difficulty sleeping. Chronic anxiety and stress may weaken the immune system and can lead to unhealthy behaviors such as overeating.

How is Anxiety Treated by Conventional Medicine?

Many patients with cancer are able to manage their anxiety and stress by increasing their sense of control through learning about their cancer and cancer treatment, practicing cognitive-behavioral techniques, and by participating in counseling and support groups.

Doctors may prescribe medication if anxiety becomes extreme, intolerable, or persists for weeks or months. Common classes of medications prescribed are benzodiazepines, azapirones, antidepressants, beta-blockers, and antihistamines.

Integrative Approaches to Anxiety

Integrative therapies can be woven into your conventional care for additional relief. A combination of integrative therapies may be required. Start with learning a therapy that you are likely to use in both acute and chronic situations. In our practice, we suggest patients begin with aromatherapy, reflexology, and visual imagery. These therapies can be administered anywhere and anytime. For example, visual imagery can be beneficial while waiting for the results of a medical test. For acute stress and anxiety, choose a therapy that can be applied immediately such as aromatherapy and visualization. If your anxiety is chronic, a routine yoga practice may provide relief. Chronic anxiety may also be helped with dietary modification or nutrition supplements. Massage therapy may be used anytime during or after treatment.

Before adding any integrative therapy to your treatment plan, speak with your doctor about the benefits and risks. A summary of risks may be found in the Introduction along with detailed instructions for the application of and considerations for each of the indicated therapies.

Integrative Medicine in Action

Patient Story
Integrative Medicine Plan for Anxiety and Stress:
Aromatherapy, Massage, and Visual Imagery.

Patient: Catherine, a 58-year old woman with metastatic melanoma experiencing anxiety.

Chief Complaint: With a history of anxiety prior to being diagnosed with cancer, Catherine's anxiety and stress levels reached an extreme level as she felt completely out of control and full of fear. She resisted joining a support group because the group environment only made her feel more stressed out.

Treatment: Still finding herself anxious even after one month of taking a benzodiazepine prescribed by her doctor, Catherine wanted to incorporate something in her daily routine that could help her manage her anxiety. She decided to set aside time for an evening bath with either Roman chamomile or rose essential oil every day. After her bath, Catherine began practicing visual imagery, which helped slow her heartbeat and prepare her for a good night's sleep. When Catherine felt particularly restless, she practiced self-massage, rubbing her ears, wrists, palms, and the bottoms of her feet.

Outcome: After just a few weeks of integrating this self-care routine, Catherine felt more at ease and started to identify feelings and situations in her life that brought on her anxiety. When Catherine noticed her anxiety levels rising, she used self-massage to stop her anxiety from getting out of control, and as a result, she was better able to go about her daily activities.

Aromatherapy

Many essential oils help us relax. Essential oils can be directly inhaled, added to a bath, or prepared as a mist to freshen a room. Consider carrying aromatherapy with you during stressful situations as you can easily use aromatherapy with the inhalation method. Aromatherapy can also help you unwind at the end of the day. Instructions for application of aromatherapy may be found in Chapter 4.

Bath: Lavender, Lemon, Roman chamomile, Rose

Diffusion/Direct inhalation: Frankincense, Lemon, Orange, Rose, Rosemary Sandalwood, Ylang ylang

Massage/Reflexology: Bergamot, Lavender, Lemon, Roman chamomile, Rose, Sandalwood

Mist: Lavender, Lemon, Orange, Roman chamomile, Rose, Rosemary, Ylang ylang

Special Applications

• Directly apply Frankincense and/or Sandalwood on acupressure point Ren 17 (Appendix A).
• Directly apply Lavender on acupressure point Yin Tang (Appendix A).

Chinese Medicine/Acupressure

Emotions can cause disruption in the flow of qi when they are sudden, severe or ongoing, and unresolved. Each emotion has a different effect on qi and subsequently presents with different symptoms. All of us experience emotional disruption in different ways. For example, when faced with news of illness we can experience a combination of anger, fear, sadness, and grief. Chinese medicine seeks to identify the primary emotion involved in order to treat what we might broadly refer to as anxiety and stress. You may feel the primary emotion most frequently, and it can dominate your reaction to stressful situations.

Symptoms of emotional imbalance are never separated from physical symptoms in Chinese medicine. Below is a description of the effect of specific emotions that can lead to anxiety and stress along with additional symptoms that they may present. Since most often we experience multiple emotions with anxiety and stress, you could combine points from several of the lists presented in this book. Acupressure can work quickly to alleviate anxiety, so you should try different points to see which ones work best for you.

Acupressure

You can use these points whenever you are experiencing anxiety or stress. You can also use them before a stressful situation to help keep you relaxed.

Most frequently used (Appendix A)
Ear Shenmen, Kid 1, Liv 3, PC 6, UB 15, Yin Tang *(stroke lightly in upward direction)*
Secondary points (Appendix A)
If you are experiencing excessive worry or overthinking, add: Liv 1, Ren 12, SP 6
If you are experiencing palpitations, add: GB 9, HT 4 to 7 (all four HT points can be stimulated together by thumb stroking down towards the wrist crease), PC 5, PC 8
If you are experiencing feelings of fear with "butterflies in the stomach," add: Kid 1, LI 4, PC 7
If accompanied by shortness of breath/chest pain/heavy sensation: HT 8, Kid 27, Ren 17

Herbal Teas

There are many different herbal teas that may be considered for relief of anxiety and stress. Some of the most commonly recommended teas are Chamomile (*Matricaria spp*), Lemon balm (*Melissa officinalis*), Linden flowers (*Tilia spp*), Oat tops, or Oatstraw (*Aveena sativa*), Passionflower (*Passiflora incarnata*), Scullcap (*Scuttellaria lateriaflora*), and Valerian (*Valeriana spp*). The teas can be sipped alone or in combination.

Typical tea combinations are provided. Instructions for tea preparation may be found in Chapter 4.

- Chamomile (1 to 2 tsp) and Passionflower (1 to 2 tsp) in 8 ounces of warm water, seep 5 to 10 minutes, and strain.
- Oatstraw or Oat tops. Seep 1/2 to 1 tsp per 32 ounces of warm water for 4 to 8 hours, and strain.
- Passionflower (1 to 2 tsp) and Linden flowers (1 to 2 tsp) in 8 ounces boiling water, seep 5 to 10 minutes, and strain.
- Skullcap (1 tsp), Passionflower (1 to 2 tsp), and Lemon balm (1 to 2 tsp) in 8 ounces of warm water, seep 5 to 10 minutes, and strain.

Homeopathy

Choose the remedy that best describes your type of anxiety. The highlighted remedies are those that are most commonly recommended, but others may also be helpful. The dosing will be different for acute and chronic anxiety. For acute anxiety begin with 30x every 2 to 4 hours, discontinue after 2 days. For chronic anxiety begin with 6x or 12x, 2 to 3 times per day. If your anxiety becomes acute, follow the dosing for acute anxiety. Discontinue when symptoms resolve.

- Aconitum. Acute states of anxiety, associated with panic attacks, anxiety associated with difficulty breathing.
- Arsenicum album. Anxiety related to fear, nervousness related to death, fear of anticipatory events.
- **Gelsemium.** Anticipatory anxiety or fear, feeling paralyzed, loss of will, fear of losing control.
- **Ignatia.** Acute states of anxiety, experiencing uncontrollable emotions.
- Phosphorous. Anxious about health, afraid of death, feel better when interacting with friends/family, nervous.
- Stramonium. Anxiety related to shock, new environments, observing an emotional event (death, disaster), violent outbursts or actions.

Massage

Massage is one of the most common therapies used to manage stress and anxiety and can be beneficial for all types of anxiety. Daily massage sessions may be particularly helpful with persistent feelings of stress or anxiety. Information on the recommended massage techniques may be found in Chapter 4.

Massage by a Caregiver

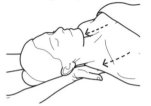

1 Have the person lie down on their back. Massage the palms of hands, upper back, in between the shoulder blades and the back of the neck, forehead, and face with petrissage motions.

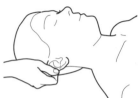

2 Gently tug the ear with your fingers.

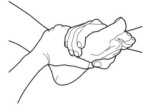

3 Massage the entire foot with particular attention to the ankles and bottom of the foot with petrissage motions (circular, squeezing, and small strokes).

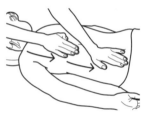

4 Have the person lie on their stomach. Massage the back while focusing on the paraspinal muscles on either side of the spine (**but not directly on the spine**) with effleurage strokes.

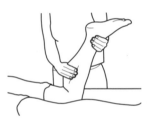

5 Massage the lower back and calves with petrissage motions (circular, squeezing, pulling, and small strokes).

Self Massage

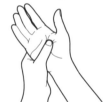

1 Gently tug your ears with your fingers.

2 With your thumb, massage each palm of your hand using friction motion.

Nutrition

Anxiety and stress can promote unhealthy dietary habits. It is easy to turn to food for comfort; however, certain foods may worsen feelings of stress and anxiety and lead to unwanted weight gain. Foods and beverages containing caffeine (coffee, chocolate, caffeinated tea, carbonated beverages, and fortified energy drinks), heavily spiced, salted, or fatty foods (Cajun-spiced, Indian, deep fried), alcohol, refined sugar (white flour breads, cookies, cakes, cereal bars with high-fructose corn syrup), and fatty snack products (chips, fried snacks) should be consumed less frequently during periods of acute stress or during the week prior to stressful procedures. If you find that your stress and anxiety increase when you eat these foods, completely avoid them during stressful periods.

Some foods may be helpful during times of high anxiety and stress and may promote calmness and relaxation. Choose foods that are aromatically pleasing and neutral (whole grains, lightly cooked vegetables (avoid vegetables served with rich sauces, excessive butter, oil, or spices), roasted or lightly sautéed poultry). Prepare

Quick Dietary Tips

• Eliminate or decrease caffeine and alcohol during periods of high stress or anxiety
• Avoid white bread, grains and pasta. Choose 100% whole grain varieties
• Be mindful of your food and environment, keep it calm and relaxed and avoid thinking about or discussing stressful topics

foods with fresh (rather than dry) herbs such as basil, parsley, cilantro, dill, and mint. Foods containing complex carbohydrates such as 100% whole wheat bread and grains, brown rice, kashi, barley, and quinoa promote feelings of relaxation and should be prioritized. Mix different whole grains for variety or combine with toppings such as toasted sesame seeds or roasted pine nuts. Add citrus dressings for variety and flavor. Include boiled (not sautéed) greens, simple salads with minimal dressings (choose olive oil-based dressings rather than creamy dressings), turkey wraps, and broth-based soups (avoid creamy soups). If you have a sweet tooth, a three ounce portion of good quality chocolate (chocolate made with at least 35% cocoa) may satisfy your sweet tooth.

Most importantly, avoid managing stress through eating. Eat meals and snacks at designated times in the day. Enjoy your meals in a relaxed environment, listening to soothing music, or dine at your favorite restaurant or at home with family and friends. Try to avoid thinking about stressful or anxiety-provoking situations during meal time.

Anxiety and stress can also suppress your immune system. Refer to the chapter on Immunosuppression to support your immune system during periods of high stress and anxiety.

Reflexology

Reflexology is one of the easiest self-remedies to apply if you are experiencing feelings of anxiety or stress. Take time to learn the points on the hands, as these can be easily stimulated before, during, or after an anxious encounter. If possible, have a caregiver stimulate foot points as you are working on your hands. Information on reflexology technique may be found in Chapter 4.

Foot Points
H: Pineal, pituitary reflexes
R: Adrenal reflexes
T: Diaphragm, heart, lung, solar plexus reflexes; rub the whole foot

Hand Points
H: Pituitary reflexes
R: Adrenal reflexes
T: Diaphragm, heart, liver, lung, solar plexus, stomach reflexes

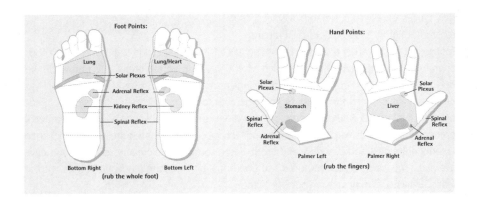

Supplements

With your doctor's approval and oversight, dietary supplements may be used to help manage symptoms of stress and anxiety. Some clinical studies have found that combining herbal or nutrition supplements with prescription medications provide a greater benefit. Certain supplements such as melatonin can interact with certain types of chemotherapy agents; corticosteroids (prednisone, hydrocortisone, dexamethasone) and anthracyclines (doxorubicin, daunorubicin) and should be avoided if you are receiving these agents.

Preoperative anxiety
• Melatonin. Oral melatonin in doses of 5 to 20 mg per day (maximum dose 20mg once per day); children 0.02mg/pound per day. Begin supplementation 2 days before procedure.

Generalized Anxiety
• Lemon balm (*Melissa officianalis*). 395 mg per day.

- Passion flower (*Passiflora incarnata*). 90mg per day. If consuming in extract form administer 45 drops per day.
- **Valerian (*Valeriana officinalis*).** 220 to 900 mg per day depending on the severity of symptoms. For restlessness: 220 mg per day. For restlessness accompanied by difficulty sleeping: 400 to 900 mg per day (refer to chapter on Insomnia).

Visual Imagery

Sit up with your back straight. Close your eyes. Start to breathe deeply. Breathe in through your nose, and out through your mouth. Allow your belly to expand as you inhale. Feel the breath going all the way down to your pelvis. Do this for five breaths.

Turn your attention to the area on your body most affected by anxiety. Is it in your chest? Your head? Your jaw? Your belly? Feel your breath filling up the area of your body that is experiencing stress or anxiety. When you exhale, envision your anxiety and stress being carried out with your breath. Continue breathing while envisioning your breath as a relaxing, peaceful, warming golden yellow sunlight. Picture this color bringing peace and harmony with every inhalation. With each exhalation, anxiety and stress is being removed. Do this for 20 to 30 breaths. Gently stop the visualization and open your eyes. If you continue to feel anxiety, repeat the process. Perform this visual exercise any time you are experiencing anxiety or stress.

Yoga

Practice breath work and yoga postures daily. In yogic theory, daily practice releases endorphins in your system and allows your breath to ease feelings of fear and anxiety. Begin with a five minute yoga routine that includes breathing exercises along with two to three poses. A beginning routine is Ujjavi breath, child's pose, and relaxation pose. As you become comfortable with this routine, add additional poses in the order of the sequence listed below always ending with child's pose and relaxation pose.

Breathing (Appendix D): Ujjayi breath, kapalabhati, alternate nostril breathing
Poses (Appendix D): Tree pose, twisting triangle pose, revolving side angle pose, straight leg seated spinal twist, cobra pose, bow pose, bridge pose, wheel pose, plough pose, child's pose, relaxation pose

Chemo Brain

What is Chemo Brain?

Chemo brain, also referred to as chemo fog, post-chemotherapy cognitive impairment, or chemotherapy-induced cognitive dysfunction, is the impairment of the brain's ability to attain, process, store, and retrieve information. People who are experiencing chemo brain may have difficulty with concentration, memory, emotions, muscle control, and may suffer from irregular sleep and wake cycles.

Chemo brain can be caused by many factors including (1) direct effects of the cancer and cancer treatment on the central nervous system; (2) side effects of some medications such as antibiotics, corticosteroids, and drugs that treat cancer related symptoms; (3) infection; (4) low red blood cell count (anemia); (5) nutrition deficiencies in iron, folic acid, and vitamin B; and (6) metabolic problems such as the decreased production of thyroid hormone. Often a combination of these factors can contribute to the development of chemo brain.

How is Chemo Brain Treated by Conventional Medicine?

Several strategies may be recommended to manage symptoms of chemo brain. These include:

- Use a daily planner to manage appointments, schedules, "to do" lists, and important dates, telephone numbers, and addresses
- Maintain daily routines
- Keep to regular sleep and exercise schedules
- Regularly perform "brain exercises" such as taking a class or word and number puzzles
- Minimize multi-tasking
- Manage stress proactively
- Attend support groups or counseling

Certain treatments may be recommended to target specific factors linked with chemo brain. For example, if chemo brain is related to anemia, erythropoietin alpha may be prescribed, and if related to nutritional deficiencies, vitamin supplementation and dietary changes may be recommended. Testing may be necessary to evaluate the full extent of symptoms (often referred to as neuropsychological testing). In some cases, medications used to treat attention deficit disorder, Alzheimer's disease, or dementia such as stimulants, cholinesterase inhibitors, antidepressants, and opiate derivates may be prescribed by your doctor.

Integrative Approaches to Chemo Brain

If you are experiencing early signs of chemo brain, consider visualization, yoga, and aromatherapy. Carry your favorite essential oil with you, and experiment with the recommended applications. If you can find a peaceful environment, follow the visualization to clear your mind. If you prefer a moving meditation, yoga can be beneficial to your mind as well as your cardiovascular system, which may also help with chemo brain. If you find that chemo brain is worse during certain periods of the day, this could be related to diet. Experiment with the dietary recommendations particularly around the time of day your symptoms are most bothersome. If you are experiencing severe symptoms of chemo brain, consider a supplement.

Before adding any integrative therapy to your treatment plan, speak with your doctor about the benefits and risks. A summary of risks may be found in the Introduction along with detailed instructions for the application of and considerations for each of the indicated therapies.

Integrative Medicine in Action

Patient Story
Integrative Medicine Plan for Chemo Brain:
Nutrition, Supplements, and Yoga.
Patient: Jessica, a 32-year old woman with breast cancer experiencing chemo brain.
Chief Complaint: Jessica noticed increased signs of forgetfulness about halfway through her chemotherapy treatments. She began to worry when the symptoms of chemo brain were impacting her everyday life. She was having trouble concentrating at work and was unable to multi-task and focus during meetings. She had little patience and attention for her children at the end of the day.
Treatment: Having had experience with yoga in the past, Jessica incorporated yoga into her daily routine by practicing pranayama breathing exercises and sun salutations upon arising in the morning, and then again two hours after dinner. Jessica adopted an anti-inflammatory diet, which included a variety of fresh, unprocessed foods and a lot of fruits, vegetables, whole grains, and nuts. She also supplemented with gingko biloba and fish oils.
Outcome: By practicing yoga, eating an anti-inflammatory diet, and supplementing with gingko biloba and fish oils, Jessica felt in control of her symptoms. She was able to focus better on her tasks at work and home. Jessica continued her integrative routine even after her chemotherapy treatments were completed, as she still experienced the benefits of this routine.

Aromatherapy

Diffuse essential oils when you need to maintain concentration to complete a defined task. You may also consider combining essential oils with reflexology and acupressure. Instructions for application of aromatherapy may be found in Chapter 4.

Diffusion/Direct inhalation: Bergamot, Lemon, Mandarin, Orange, Peppermint, Tangerine.
Special Applications
• Directly inhale Frankincense and Sandalwood. Then, directly apply Frankincense and/or Sandalwood to acupressure point DU 20, and Yin Tang (Appendix A) and massage along the base of the skull (refer to the massage section in this chapter).
• Directly apply any of the essential oils listed above to the foot reflexology points listed in this section that are directed at the toes (refer to the reflexology section in this chapter).

Chinese Medicine/Acupressure

According to Chinese medicine, the brain is referred to as the Sea of Marrow. Many of the attributes ascribed to the brain in the west are the result of proper functioning of several different organ systems. In Chinese medical theory, chemotherapy and radiation put strain on the entire body and, as a result, the functioning of the organs responsible for memory and mental clarity may become impaired. For chemo brain, Chinese medicine focuses on treating the associated symptoms. For instance, acupoints will target poor memory, inability to focus, and mental fatigue.

Acupressure
Most frequently used (Appendix A)
DU 20, Kid 3, Si Chen Cong, ST 36
Secondary points (Appendix A)
• HT 7, Kid 7, SJ 4, ST 40, Tai Yang, UB 1, UB 10, Yin Tang

Herbal Teas

While you are experiencing symptoms of chemo brain, choose herbal tea over coffee, and drink the tea throughout the day especially when symptoms are most intense. Breathe in the aroma as you are drinking the tea. Instructions for tea preparation may be found in Chapter 4.

- Citrus. Choose from any citrus flavor: orange, grapefruit, lemon, lime, or tangerine. Citrus teas are usually very palatable and the strength of the tea will vary by individual. Use 1 to 4 tsp of any citrus tea in 8 ounces of hot water, seep for 5 to 10 minutes, strain.
- Peppermint (*Mentha piperita*). 1 to 2 tsp in 6 to 8 ounces of hot water, seep for 10 minutes, strain.
- Rosemary (*Rosmarinus officinalis*). 1 to 2 tsp in 6 to 8 ounces of boiling water, seep for 10 to 15 minutes, strain.

Homeopathy

Begin with the remedy(s) that is most closely associated with your symptoms. Start with a dose of 30c, 2 to 4 times per day for 4 to 6 weeks. If symptoms resolve, discontinue supplementation. If symptoms are still present, but have reduced in intensity, begin a dose of 6c or 12c for 6 to 8 weeks.

- Anacardium. Impaired memory, absent mindedness, dementia.
- Avena Sativa. Nervous exhaustion, exhaustion relating to illness or excess work, difficulty focusing and retaining information.
- Baryta carb. Loss of memory, mental weakness, indecision, low confidence, confusion and disorientation.
- Conium. Weakening of memory, body, and mind; unable to comprehend and concentrate for sustained periods of time, forgetfulness.
- Lycopodium. Weak memory, confused thoughts, frequently spells or writes incorrect words; unable to read own writing; poor concentration; confused thought.
- Phosphoric Acid. Mental and physical exhaustion, difficulty carrying out a thought, impaired memory and comprehension, difficulty finding words "too tired to think".

Massage

Massage is often considered a relaxing technique; however, the massage technique recommended for chemo brain is more invigorating. Self massage works locally to stimulate the brain, and can supplement massage by a caregiver. Self massage can be applied throughout the day and any time you feel mentally tired or are having difficulty concentrating. Information on the recommended massage techniques may be found in Chapter 4.

Massage by a Caregiver

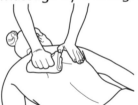

1 Rigorously massage the body with a dry or slightly wet washcloth or loofa without the use of cream or oil. This method is called skin brushing. It invigorates the circulation and stimulates the nerves that send information from the skin to the brain.

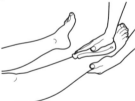

2 Start on top of one foot and move toward the knee. Press deeply enough so that there is a sensation of pressure and the skin turns slightly red. If you experience pain, or breaking the skin, lighten your touch.

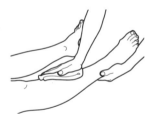

3 Massage up the front of the leg to the knee.

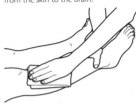

4 Repeat the massage on the inside of the ankle up to the knee and then repeat again from the outside of the ankle up to the knee.

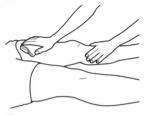

5 Begin pressing the washcloth or loofa from the knee to the groin (upper front of the thigh), on the inside of the thigh up to the groin area and then on the outside of the thigh from the knee to the hip area. Repeat this technique on the other thigh.

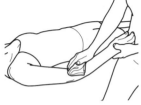

6 Begin this process on the hands and arms. Start from the top of wrist and brush up to the elbow. You may have to lighten your pressure on the inside or palm side of the arm, as it is more sensitive than the outside.

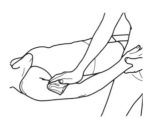

7 Begin this technique from the elbow to the shoulder on the outside of the arm and then from the elbow to the shoulder on the inside of the arm up to the armpit.

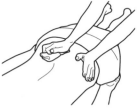

8 After the limbs have been massaged, go the buttocks and use upward motions on each side.

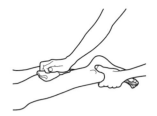

9 Repeat this process from the heel up the back of the leg to the back of the knee.

Self Massage

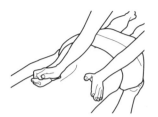

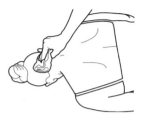

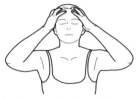

10 Repeat the process on the lower back, particularly in the area overlying the kidneys which is where the lowest ribs overlie the lower back.

11 Apply the skin brushing motion on the whole back starting from the lower back up to the neck and shoulder area.

12 Then brush up the back of the neck. Avoid the front or throat area.

13 Repeat this entire process 2-3 times.

Brush your scalp with your fingers. Your fingers will feel like a brush or comb. Start from the forehead area and move your fingers to the back of the head. Do several passes with your fingers until you have covered the entire head area.

Nutrition

Changing your diet may help relieve the fog associated with chemo brain. Small changes in your diet may also improve concentration and attention. Choose high fiber, low glycemic foods (refer to Appendix E, F), add small amounts of protein to each meal or snack, and eat at regular times each day. Most importantly, avoid overeating by choosing small portions. This is vital to preventing mental fog and decreased alertness.

Begin with these simple food substitutions and strategies

- Choose breakfast cereals made with oats, barley, and bran.
- Choose breads with 100% whole grains, stone-ground flour, or sourdough.
- Avoid white and sweet potatoes.
- Eat one fiber-rich fruit once or twice each day e.g. apples, fresh or dried apricots, cherries, grapefruit, orange, peach, pear, plum, raspberries, strawberries, blueberries, figs.
- Try one nutrient-rich vegetable once or twice each day e.g. broccoli, Brussels sprouts, kale, asparagus, cabbage, okra, turnips, mushrooms, spinach, tomato, zucchini, cauliflower, celery, cucumber, green beans, green pepper, dark colored salad leaves, bok choy, mustard greens.
- Choose basmati, wild, or doongara rice instead of white rice.
- Cook pasta or quinoa *al dente*.
- Add vinaigrette dressing to salads; avoid creamy dressings.
- Choose a brain boosting snack a few times per day such as cheese; nut butters; avocado with whole wheat crackers; dried beans; yogurt flavored with berries or agave nectar; celery sticks topped with nut butter or cream cheese.

- Rosemary has long been revered for helping to boost memory. Season chicken, fish, or vegetables with fresh or dried rosemary.
- Avoid "super size" portions, instead eat to the point of satisfaction.
- When dining out, request adult entrées in child-size portions or ask that half of your entrée be served, and the other half packaged for take away. A guide to portion control is provided in Appendix G.

Quick Dietary Tips

- Combine protein and carbohydrate in both meals and snacks
- Monitor portion sizes
- Avoid overeating
- Choose foods low on the glycemic index

Reflexology

Combine reflexology with self massage to improve mental clarity. Stimulate the points throughout the day or when you begin to experience symptoms of chemo brain. Information on reflexology technique may be found in Chapter 4.

Foot Points
F: Brain reflex on all the tips of the toes
H: Pineal, Pituitary reflexes
R: Adrenal reflexes
T: Spinal reflex; neck and shoulder line

Hand Points
F: Brain reflex on all the tips of the fingers
H: Pineal, pituitary reflexes
T: Spinal reflex

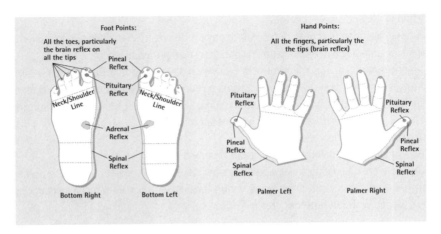

Supplements

Supplements can be beneficial for chemo brain; however, many of the suggested supplements can interact with chemotherapy or are contraindicated in medical conditions common to patients with cancer. If your doctor approves the use of a supplement, try it for 2–3 months. If relief is not obtained within two to three months, discontinue and consider a different supplement or complementary therapy.

- Brahmi *(Bacopa monnieri)*. This herbal remedy has its roots in Ayurvedic medicine. Brahmi has been traditionally prescribed for difficulties with memory and concentration. The dose is 300 mg per day for 12 weeks.
- **Essential fatty acids (Fish oils).** 4 to 6 grams per day of a mixture of eicosapentanoic acid (EPA) and docosahexaenoic acid (DHA). Choose supplements that provide approximately 70% EPA/30% DHA. **Fish oils may be contraindicated if you have problems with blood clotting and/or if you taking a blood thinner.**
- **Gingko biloba/Panax ginseng.** Gingko is one of the most widely used supplements for difficulties with concentration and memory. The dose of gingko is 120 to 240 mg per day. The combination of gingko with panax ginseng (3 to 4 grams per day for 12 weeks) or rhodiola may provide improved relief. **Panax ginseng should be avoided if you have a hormone-sensitive cancer such as breast or prostate cancer.** Gingko can interfere with many classes of drugs.
- *Rhodiola (Rhodiola rosea).* The dose is 340 to 500 mg per day for 4 weeks. Start with the lowest dose, and if benefits are not observed within 4 weeks, increase as tolerated.

Visual Imagery

You will get the most benefit from this visual imagery exercise if you are sitting with your spine straight.

Close your eyes and take several deep breaths. As you inhale, the belly should expand or push out. When you exhale, imagine the breath moving up the spine from the lower back all the way up through the back of the head, around the top of the head, down the forehead, and out your nose. Breathe in, filling the front of your body from your nose to your throat to the chest, down to your belly. As the air enters your body, your chest and belly should expand outward as if a balloon is being filled with air. When you exhale, imagine the air moving up the back through the lower lumbar area up the spine through the back of the head, around to the front of your head and out your nose. Repeat this process five times. Feel this breathing process awaken your body.

Now, keeping your eyes closed, imagine a bright yellow beam of light pouring in through the top of your head and filling up the space behind your eyes and inside your head. Imagine this yellow light invigorating your brain cells. Imagine the light of the sun inside your head. Imagine this sunlight drying up what you can imagine to be fog inside your head. As the yellow light fills your head, imagine your concentration getting clearer. The more you imagine this light entering into your head, the more the fog is burned off, like the sun on the morning dew. Your concentration improves. Hold this image for a few minutes.

Now tell yourself that this beam of invigorating yellow light also improves your focus, your memory, alertness, fatigue and clarity. Continue to feel and see with your mind's eye this yellow light invigorating your brain. Hold that feeling. Tell yourself, either silently or aloud:

> "Every time I imagine this yellow light coming into the top of my head I become more alert, and my memory and concentration improve."

While visualizing the invigorating light, repeat this sentence three times. When you have completed this process three times, gently bring your focus back into the room.

When you go about your day, you can use this visualization as a quick reminder that this yellow light brings about clarity and alertness.

Repeat as necessary.

Yoga

Sun salutation is a short yoga routine that can wake up the mind and body. Practice this routine in the morning to bring energy and awareness to your day. The headstand posture is an advanced posture and should be practiced with caution. Practice the breathing technique throughout the day.

Breathing (Appendix D): Ujjayi breath, alternate nostril breathing
Poses (Appendix D): Sun salutation, standing forward bend, headstand, relaxation pose

Constipation

What is Constipation?

Constipation, a common side effect of cancer therapy, is a condition when bowel movements become infrequent and stools become too hard, small, dry, or difficult to pass. Symptoms of constipation include abdominal pain, bloating, cramping, and painful bowel movements. Constipation may be the result of chemotherapy treatments, a tumor putting pressure on the bowel, pain, anxiety, and medications, such as certain pain medications. Lifestyle habits can also contribute to constipation; these include ignoring the urge to pass stool, decreased fluid intake, low or decreased dietary fiber, inadequate movement or exercise, and stress.

How is Constipation Treated by Conventional Medicine?

Conventional medical practitioners typically manage constipation by monitoring bowel function, promoting a regular schedule for toileting, and prescribing medications such as stool softeners (docusate sodium) or laxatives (senna, magnesium citrate). Stool softeners will soften hard stools, whereas laxatives promote gastrointestinal movement. Rectal administration of enemas or suppositories should be avoided if you have low platelet counts, low white blood cell counts, or sores of the rectum or colon from cancer and its treatment as this can lead to the development of anal fissures or abscesses, which can be an entry route for infection.

Integrative Approaches to Constipation

Integrative medicine relies on multiple theories to managing constipation. We often recommend dietary changes followed by massage, reflexology, or yoga to promote movement in the intestines. Start with the dietary changes as these may take some time and attention. Once the dietary changes are mastered, begin with an additional therapy. If physical movement is difficult, choose massage or acupressure. You may also add aromatherapy to any of the touch therapies.

If constipation is an expected side effect of your cancer therapy, consider supplements or herbal teas to help prevent constipation from occurring. Supplements can become habit-forming, so only use during times at high risk for constipation. Avoid using supplements for chronic constipation. Instead, choose dietary change, exercise, and massage.

Before adding any integrative therapy to your treatment plan, speak with your doctor about the benefits and risks. A summary of risks may be found in the Introduction along with detailed instructions for the application of and considerations for each of the indicated therapies.

Integrative Medicine in Action

Patient Story
Integrative Medicine Plan for Constipation:
Nutrition and Yoga.
Patient: Lily, a 24-year old woman with Acute Lymphoblastic Leukemia experiencing constipation.
Chief Complaint: Since being diagnosed with leukemia, Lily has had short periods of constipation due to chemotherapy that generally resolved on its own. But now, after a few weeks of taking an anxiety medication, Lily's constipation has become unbearable. Her stool is dry, and she is experiencing unmanageable bloating. Despite her anxiety medication making her constipation worse, Lily is afraid to stop taking it.
Treatment: After learning about ways to change her diet, Lily modified her daily food intake. For breakfast, she switched to an oat bran cereal topped with raspberries, blueberries, and one tablespoon of whole flax seeds. She made sure to avoid fast food at lunch and dinner and instead chose meals that were high in both soluble and insoluble fiber. She incorporated pearl barley, lentils, and spinach into her meals. Throughout the day, she ate walnuts and drank hot lemon juice. She also drank 1/2 to 1 glass of water every hour while awake. Every morning, Lily set aside time to practice the yogic breathing exercises (ujjayi breath and kapalabhati). When she had enough energy, she followed the yoga breathing with yoga twisting and backbending postures.
Outcome: Over the period of a month, Lily slowly began to feel relief. Her bowel movements became more regular, and her stool became softer. She also felt her anxiety was more under control.

Aromatherapy

Aromatherapy can be beneficial when combined with massage over the belly. Instructions for application of aromatherapy may be found in Chapter 4.

Compress/Direct Application/Massage: Black pepper, Fennel, Ginger, Peppermint, Roman chamomile. Compress should be applied to the lower belly.
Special Applications
• Directly apply any of the essential oils listed above on acupressure points LI 4 and ST 25 (Appendix A).
• Directly apply Black pepper essential oil to large intestine foot and hand reflexology points (refer to the reflexology section in this chapter).
• Perform abdominal massage using essential oil blend of Black pepper, Peppermint, and Roman chamomile in a 1:1:1: ratio (refer to the massage section in this chapter).

Chinese Medicine/Acupressure

Constipation refers to a decrease in the frequency of bowel movements or to difficulty in defecation due to dry and impacted stool. The causes of constipation are many. Examples include hot or cold accumulation, deficiency of fluids, and/or qi and qi stagnation. Heat accumulation and deficiency of fluids in the intestines can cause body fluids to be consumed and dryness to develop; therefore, there will not be sufficient lubrication for proper movement. Cold accumulation can cause stool to become impacted by inhibiting the flow of qi in the intestines. Qi stagnation is largely caused by emotional stress leading to a disruption in the natural flow of qi in the intestines. Deficiency of qi resulting from illness or weakness will make it difficult for the peristalsis of the intestine to discharge the stool.

Acupressure
Most frequently used (Appendix A)
SJ 6, ST 25, ST 37
Secondary points (Appendix A)
If accompanied by feverishness, dry mouth, and foul breath, add: LI 4, LI 11, ST 44
If accompanied by pain that is relieved with warmth and cold limbs, add: DU 4, Ren 4, Ren 6
If accompanied by abdominal distention with frequent belching, add: GB 34, Ren 12
If accompanied by weakness and fatigue after bowel movement, add: Ren 6, SP 6, ST 36

Herbal Teas

Herbal teas are most effective when consumed warm or hot. Honey or agave nectar, generally added to enhance flavor, can also promote intestinal movement. Drink herbal teas around the time of your normal bowel movement. If you do not have a bowel movement at approximately the same time every day, choose a time that best fits your schedule. Instructions for tea preparation may be found in Chapter 4.

- Cascara Sagrada (*Rhamnus purshiana*). 1 tsp to 8 ounces of boiling water, seep for 10 minutes, and strain.
- Senna (*Cassia species*). 1/2 to 1 tsp to 8 ounces of warm water, seep for 10 minutes, and strain.

Homeopathy

Choose the remedy most closely associated with your symptoms of constipation. For acute constipation, begin with a dose of 12x, every hour for a maximum of 4 doses per day. If relief is not obtained, increase the dose to 30x. Discontinue with a bowel movement. If relief is not obtained within 24 hours, consider a higher dose, increased repetition, or another remedy. For chronic constipation, choose a dose of 6x, 2 to 3 times per day for a maximum of 2 to 3 weeks. Discontinue once symptoms resolve.

- Alumina. Severe straining leading to a soft stool.
- **Bryonia.** Little urge to pass stools, stools are large, hard, and dry.
- Lycopodium. Little urge to pass stools, no stool passed, pain accompanies the urge for a bowel movement, desire for sweet foods.
- Natrum mur. Dry stools, passed infrequently, associated with bleeding, pain, and soreness.
- Nux Vomica. Frequent urge to pass stools, small amounts of stool passed, history of chronic laxative use.

Massage

Massage can be especially beneficial in promoting gut movement. Massage as needed throughout the day, no more than four times in a 24-hour period. Information on the recommended massage techniques may be found in Chapter 4.

Massage by a Caregiver

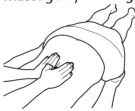 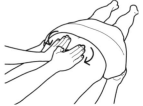 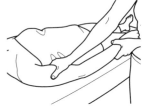

1 Have the person lie on their stomach. Massage the lower back with effleurage strokes.

2 Massage the sacrum (triangle shaped bone on the bottom of the spine) and right above the hip bones with petrissage circular motions.

3 Have the person lie on their back. Massage the arms starting from the wrist up to the shoulder with petrissage squeezing motion.

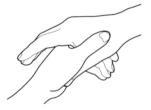

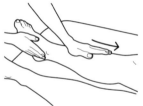

4 Massage the web of the hand between the forefinger and the thumb with circular friction motion.

5 Massage the outer side of the shin bone on the lower leg with effleurage strokes.

Self Massage

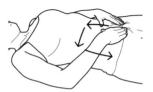

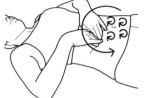

1 Massage the lower left side of the belly starting at the hip bone and moving up the left side under the ribs with small, circular petrissage motions.

2 Massage across the upper belly under the ribs moving towards the right side with small, circular petrissage motions.

3 Massage down the right side of the body ending at the right hip bone with small, circular petrissage motions.

4 Massage the lower belly around the belly button in a clockwise direction with small, circular petrissage motions.

5 Massage the entire lower belly with petrissage motions, as if you are kneading dough.

Nutrition

Proper nutrition is essential for the prevention and management of constipation. Specific dietary patterns can decrease the frequency and duration of constipation by softening stools and stimulating movement of the bowel.

Foods containing high levels of insoluble fiber and foods high in caffeine such as coffee or dark chocolate (at least 50% cocoa) can promote gut movement. Drinking warm liquids may be especially beneficial if taken just prior to your usual time for a bowel movement.

Intake of olive oil, honey, and nectars are also recommended. Historically, these foods are thought to "lubricate" the gut, thereby promoting bowel activity.

Quick Dietary Tips

Fiber is the most widely promoted dietary antidote for constipation. Fiber is categorized as insoluble and soluble. Insoluble fiber is best for decreased gut movement, whereas soluble fiber acts more as a stool softener. In the case of decreased movement with hard stools, a combination of both insoluble and soluble fiber would be most appropriate.

• Drink liquids throughout the day, particularly hot liquids (laxative teas) and warmed fruit juices (prune, apple, pear, syrup of figs, and black cherry are good choices)
• Increase water intake
• Add insoluble fiber to your diet. Increase the insoluble fiber in your diet in 5 to 8 gram increments per day. Aim for a daily total fiber goal of 25 to 30 grams per day

When increasing the fiber in your diet, it is crucial to increase your fluid intake. Strive for at least three to six, 8 ounce glasses of water each day. Increased dietary fiber will only be effective if water is increased at the same time. If you are taking laxatives, avoid foods high in soluble fiber until you experience movement in your bowels.

Food Remedies

• Choose 2 to 3 foods high in *insoluble* fiber each day. These include figs, raspberries, blackberries, pears, cranberries, cooked spinach, peas, cooked green beans, okra, sunflower seeds, pearl barley, and most types of beans (Appendix C).
• Choose 2 to 3 "lubricating" foods each day. Experiment with spinach, asparagus, sweet potato, papaya, banana, honey, pear, prune, peach, apple, apricot, walnut (1 to 2 tablespoons per day), pine nut, black sesame seed, coconut, almond, soy, carrot, cauliflower, beet, okra, and seaweed. According to TCM principles, these foods "lubricate" the bowels.
• Avoid or limit foods that may cause bloating and gas such as raw cabbage, beans, and carbonated beverages. The inclusion of these foods will depend on your previous and current intake of them. If these foods are new to your dietary regimen, do not introduce them during periods of constipation. Beans can be beneficial for the prevention of constipation but may aggravate bloating or gas if constipation is more severe.
• Choose a breakfast cereal that is a high-bran (oat bran) cereal, 1/2 cup to 1 1/2 cups each day.
• Experiment with boiled greens. Boiled collard greens or dandelion greens sprinkled with olive oil and lemon may promote gut movement.
• Add 1 to 2 tablespoons of whole flax seeds (not flax meal) to any food or dish such as cereal, any baked-good mix, smoothies, casseroles, or yogurt. Flax seeds promote gut movement.

• Drink hot lemon juice throughout the day and prior to your usual time for a bowel movement. Squeeze 1/2 to 1 lemon in 6 to 8 ounces of warm water. You can also choose warm prune, apple, pear, or black cherry juice.

Reflexology

Reflexology may be used throughout the day as needed. Information on reflexology technique may be found in Chapter 4.

Foot Points

H: Ileocecal valve, sigmoid colon reflexes
R: Adrenal, gallbladder reflexes
T: Diaphragm, large intestine, liver, lumbar/sacrum, small intestine reflexes

Hand Points

T: Large intestine, lumbar/sacrum, small intestine reflexes

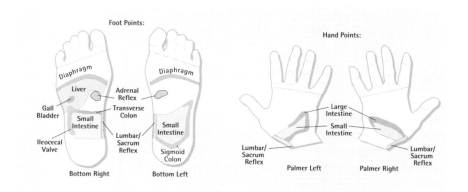

Supplements

Similar to prescribed medications, supplements can be habit forming and are not indicated for long term use. If you have not experienced relief with other complementary therapies or if you are at high risk for the development of constipation, work with your doctor to choose a supplement that might be right for you. The supplements listed below are available in either powder or capsule form. If you choose a powder form, begin with black or blond psyllium. You can mix these powders into a fruit smoothie or into a liquid. If you prefer a capsule, choose cascara, senna, or dandelion root.

- **Black or Blond psyllium.** Black psyllium seeds act in the same manner as laxatives. Blond psyllium has properties similar to insoluble fiber and is indicated for both constipation and diarrhea. The recommended dose for black or blond psyllium is 10 to 30 grams per day. Start low (5 grams per day) and increase as needed. The effective dose will depend on the severity of your constipation and how much fiber is already a part of your diet. As you increase insoluble fiber in your diet, decrease supplementation with psyllium. Be careful if combining with strong laxatives such as cascara, senna, or rhubarb. Fluid intake must be increased with intake of black or blond psyllium.
- Castor Oil. Traditionally promoted as a natural gut "lubricant" or "moistener," 1 to 3 tbsp per day, as needed.
- **Dandelion root, Senna, and Cascara Sagrada.** These laxative herbs act as stimulants and are listed in the order of their strength, from mild to strong. These are often combined with psyllium to promote movement, while adding bulk to the stool.
  - ➤ Dandelion root (*Taraxacum officinale*): 500 mg, 1 to 3 times per day.
  - ➤ Senna (*Cassia species*): In the United States, products are Senokot® and Ex-Lax®. Your doctor or pharmacist can help you determine the appropriate dose. Doses are typically in the range of 18 to 35 mg per day (max dose 35 mg per day).
  - ➤ Cascara Sagrada (*Rhamnus purshiana*): 425 mg per day, 1 to 2 times per day.

Yoga

According to yogic theory, the occurrence of constipation is correlated with the tone of the abdominal and rectal/anal muscles. The following yoga sequence should be performed every morning to tone these muscles. Begin with breathing and the first three poses. Add additional poses until the vinyasa is completed in the order listed. You can perform these exercises as much as needed until relief is obtained.

Breathing (Appendix D): Ujjayi breath, kapalabhati
Poses (Appendix D): Triangle pose, twisting triangle pose, revolving side angle pose, downward facing dog pose, standing forward bend, child's pose, cobra pose, bow pose, camel pose, shoulderstand, plough pose, supine twist, supine knee squeeze, relaxation pose

Depression

What is Depression?

Depression is often described as a feeling of gloom, emptiness, numbness, or despair and can exist on a continuum of emotional responses from slight mood changes to severe depression. Depression may be part of a grief response to a cancer diagnosis or cancer treatment and occurs quite often, with at least one in four patients with cancer experiencing clinical depression. A history of depression before the cancer diagnosis, uncontrolled pain, nutritional problems, hyperthyroidism, hypothyroidism, and increased physical discomfort all contribute to the experience of depression.

If feelings of sadness or grief last a minimum of two weeks and are present on most days for a long time or interfere with daily activities, further evaluation is often necessary. Symptoms of depressed mood, especially if associated with a loss of interest in daily activities, warrant medical supervision. Treatment for depression may be especially beneficial for patients with four of more of the following symptoms:

- Trouble sleeping (difficulty falling asleep, waking early, sleeping too much)
- Eating problems (eating too little or too much, with associated weight loss or gain)
- Fatigue or feelings of decreased energy
- Mood changes such as feelings of irritability
- Feelings of worthlessness or hopelessness
- Thoughts of self-harm
- Preoccupation with death
- Difficulty with memory or concentration
- Social withdrawal
- Crying spells

How is Depression Treated by Conventional Medicine?

Management of depression may include counseling or psychotherapy, behavior therapy, cancer education sessions, and support groups. Speaking with a clergy member may be helpful for some people. Major depression may also be treated with a combination of counseling and antidepressant medications. Decisions about which antidepressant will depend on your symptoms, previous exposure to antidepressant medications, and the possible side effects or interactions associated with the antidepressant. Most antidepressants must be taken for three to six weeks before relief is experienced.

Integrative Approaches to Depression

The integrative approach to depression will depend on the duration and severity of your symptoms. For newly diagnosed depression, lifestyle changes including yoga, nutrition, and guided visualization may be beneficial. Various essential oils can be easily diffused into a room for an uplifting effect. Asking your spouse, a friend, or a caregiver to make similar lifestyle changes will provide support and make new habits easier to adopt. Supplements are sometimes used for treatment of depression; however, many supplements recommended for depression interfere with chemotherapy drugs. **Speak with your doctor before beginning any supplement.**

Before adding any integrative therapy to your treatment plan, speak with your doctor about the benefits and risks. A summary of risks may be found in the Introduction along with detailed instructions for the application of and considerations for each of the indicated therapies.

Integrative Medicine in Action

Patient Story

Integrative Medicine Plan for Depression:
Visual Imagery and Yoga.

Patient: Damian, a 45-year old man with lung cancer experiencing depression.

Chief Complaint: Although Damian recovered fairly well from the initial shock of his diagnosis, during his first course of chemotherapy he began to lose his appetite, experienced difficulty sleeping, and was engulfed by a sense of hopelessness. He avoided seeing his friends, and refused to answer his phone. Damian was also finding it difficult to get to his doctor's appointments.

Treatment: Damian's oncologist identified his symptoms of depression and encouraged him to join a bi-weekly hospital-led yoga class for patients. He found the yoga class provided him with social support and the yoga helped improve his energy level. Damian also learned about visual imagery. If he felt a wave of depression coming on, he would practice yoga and breathing exercises, especially alternate nostril technique. By practicing on a daily basis, he began to have a sense of control and hope.

Outcome: Damian was better able to manage his sense of hopelessness through visual imagery. After four weeks of a consistent yoga routine, he noticed the intensity of his depression had diminished.

Aromatherapy

Combining aromatherapy with acupressure or reflexology or diffusing essential oils in a room can lift up one's mood. Using essential oils with a massage at times during the day when you are feeling especially low may also provide some relief. Instructions for application of aromatherapy may be found in Chapter 4.

Diffusion/Direct inhalation: Bergamot, Frankincense, Grapefruit, Lavender, Orange, Peppermint, Rose.

Massage: Bergamot, Lavender, Rose.

Special Applications

- Directly apply Frankincense and/or Lavender and/or Rose on acupressure point Ren 17 (Appendix A).
- Directly apply Bergamot and/or Orange and/or Grapefruit on acupressure point ST 36 (Appendix A).
- Directly inhale Frankincense and Peppermint. Then, directly apply Peppermint at acupressure point DU 20 (Appendix A) and massage along base of the skull.
- Diffuse Orange in your room as part of your morning routine before leaving your home.

Chinese Medicine/Acupressure

Chinese medicine has many classifications for symptoms associated with depression. Anger, sadness, lack of motivation, and/or feelings of despair are each treated somewhat differently. Individual emotions are either a result of a disruption in the qi dynamic or a cause of the disruption (refer to Anxiety and Stress). Since it is very common to experience a combination of these emotions during cancer treatment, it can be helpful to determine which emotion is dominant and then to choose the most appropriate acupressure point prescription.

Acupressure

Most frequently used (Appendix A)

DU 20, Liv 3, Ren 17, Yin Tang

Secondary points (Appendix A)

If associated with anger, irritability, and moodiness, add: LI 4, Liv 2

If associated with sadness and grief and/or weak voice and frequent weeping, add: HT 7, LU 1, LU 3, Ren 17, ST 36, UB 13

If associated with feelings of despair, including inability to get out of bed, add: Kid 3, Kid 6, Kid 7, UB 23

Herbal Teas

Herbal teas may be used to help improve one's mood. Instructions for tea preparation may be found in Chapter 4.

• Chai. Chai tea is infused with spices that are thought to boost mood. This tea may be purchased ready-to-mix into warm or hot water. Sip throughout the day as needed.

Homeopathy

Homeopathy may help relieve your symptoms of depression. Clinical studies have found individualized homeopathic remedies can be beneficial in managing depression. Choose the remedies that best describe your symptoms. If you have a history of depression or are taking medications for depression, consider consultation with a homeopathic practitioner for an individualized prescription. Begin with a dose of 12cc or 30cc once per day as needed.

• *Ignatia.* Most frequently recommended remedy for depression. This remedy is typically used when fluctuating moods and difficulty controlling emotions are present.
• Nat mur. Deep emotional wounds; good for chronic depression.
• Phosphoric Acid. Apathetic, indifferent, listless, weak.
• Sepia. Overwhelmed, tired, sad, weeping, emotionally closed.

Massage

Whole body massage can invigorate the mind and relax the body. Not only are endorphins released, but massage can also reconnect us to others. Whole body massage promotes relaxation and reduces stress therapy helping with some of the symptoms associated with depression. Self massage is not the optimal therapy for depression. Information on the recommended massage techniques may be found in Chapter 4.

Massage by a Caregiver

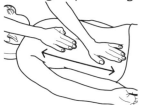

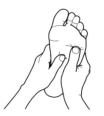

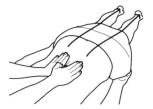

1 Massage the whole body using effleurage, petrissage, and friction strokes as indicated in the Introduction.

2 Focus on the palms of the hands and the feet using small circular petrissage motions.

3 Focus massage on the upper back, mid-back, buttocks, legs, and feet using long effleurage strokes.

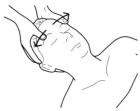

4 Finish with the neck (particularly under the skull and back of the head), ears, head, and face (particularly the frontalis muscle of the forehead and temples) using small petrissage strokes.

Nutrition

Dietary change is a component of an integrative approach for management of psychological health and well-being. Certain types of food may be triggers for an assortment of emotions. For example, refined sugar can cause feelings of fatigue and decreased mental acuity; whereas, caffeine and alcohol can either increase mental sharpness and energy or promote feelings of depression. Saturated fat can lead to satisfaction and comfort; however, excess intake may lead to fatigue.

The link between nutrition and mental health is thought to be due to nutrients found in certain types of foods that contain compounds needed to form neurotransmitters. Neurotransmitters are biochemical compounds that are always in the body and can make us feel happiness, joy, anxiety, or sadness. By changing your diet, you can increase your exposure to the types of foods that promote feelings of wellness, and decrease your intake of foods that promote fatigue, mental drain, and depression.

For dietary change to be beneficial, strict adherence to **two basic dietary strategies** is necessary. First, you should choose foods high in Omega 3s and include them in every meal. Second, choose foods low on the glycemic index (Appendix E). To the best of your ability, avoid foods low in Omega 3s and foods with a high glycemic index. As always, monitor portion sizes and avoid overeating.

Food Remedies

- Keep food selection diverse. Avoid monotonous meals.
- Engage the senses with food aromas; explore new seasonings and food ethnicities.
- Limit Caffeine. Caffeine can be a "pick-me-up," but can also have a depressant effect. Limit your caffeine intake to one cup of caffeinated drink per day. Substitute tea, flavored or non-flavored seltzer, or water.
- Experiment with coconut milk, fresh coconut, or shredded coconut at any time during the day.
- Flax meal should be added to **at least** one meal per day. Flax meal can be added to cereal, yogurt, cake or bread-mixes.

Quick Dietary Tips

- Consume foods naturally rich in Omega 3s everyday including salmon, sardines, sea bass, nuts (cashews, almond, macadamia), and flax meal. Many foods are fortified with Omega 3s such as eggs, breakfast cereals, granola or protein snack bars, waffles, and pasta
- Emphasize diversity in food selection
- Choose foods that are low on the glycemic index

Supplements

Dietary supplements may be beneficial for depression, as several clinical trials have shown antidepressant effects. Benefits from supplementation will vary and are based on prior and current use of antidepressant medications and the type symptoms being experienced. **Use of supplements for depression during cancer treatment is complex, as interactions with chemotherapy agents may occur. You and your doctor can decide if supplementation is right for your clinical condition.**

- **Eicosapentaenoic Acid (EPA).** 1 gram, 2 times per day along with conventional antidepressant medications. Benefits are usually seen within 3 weeks of treatment.
- Folic Acid. 500 micrograms to 50 mg for 2 to 6 months along with conventional antidepressant medications. This supplement may work best in patients with low blood

folate levels. This may not be beneficial in patients with normal folate levels. It should not be taken along with the chemotherapy drug, methotrexate.

• **S–Adenosylmethionine (SAMe).** 1600 mg per day. Beneficial effects have been observed within 4 to 8 weeks. Intravenous SAMe has been observed to work much faster; however, this can only be administered by a medical doctor.

• Saffron. 30 milligrams for 6 weeks. Small clinical studies have shown antidepressant effects.

• **St John's Wort** (*Hypericum perforatum*). 300 mg, 3 times per day. St. John's Wort has been found to have similar effectiveness to some of the prescription drugs for depression. Beneficial effects are experienced after 4 to 12 weeks of administration. **St. John's Wort can interfere with many chemotherapy drugs and should not be used without consultation and approval by your doctor.**

Visual Imagery

Sit in a comfortable position with your back straight. Start breathing slowly and gently into your body. When your body feels sufficiently relaxed with deep breathing, start to imagine a ball of white light hovering above your head. See that ball as a brilliant white light. Know that the ball of brilliant white light is the light of emotional healing. When you have a full and strong image of the ball of light, see it slowly descending into your body through the top of your head. Feel the warmth and see the light inside your head. Imagine this light is filling your sinuses, your eyes, your brain, your mouth, your nose. Feel the comfort of the white light.

That light now grows and continues to descend into your throat. Feel your throat open up as the light fills the area. The light now grows to encompass your shoulders, and then travels down your arms to your elbows, your forearms, your wrists, your palms and into all the fingers. This light is now in your head, throat, neck, shoulders, arms, and hands. See this beautiful, brilliant white light filling up the chest, getting rid of all feelings of despair. Feel that light as joy. Feel it move down to the diaphragm and feel and see it open up the area. You can now take a bigger and deeper breath because this light is filling you with joy and warmth.

The light now moves down to the belly and pelvis. Feel it revitalizing all your cells along the way as it moves down your body. Now see the light moving down your thighs, knees, legs, ankles, feet, and toes. This light is the light of hope, the light of joy. Stay with this image as long as you can. If you lose the image, take a deep breath and refocus. Repeat to yourself: This light I see and feel is the light of joy.

Repeat as necessary.

Yoga

Practice breath work and yoga postures daily. This combination will help release endorphins (compounds in the body that make us feel happy) and will allow your breath to ease feelings of sadness. Begin by breathing deeply and focus on the sounds of your inhalation and exhalation. Allow your mind to take you to an uplifting place. Allow your mind to take you to a safe place.

Breathing (Appendix D): Ujjayi breath, kapalabhati, alternate nostril breathing
Poses to increase energy level (Appendix D): Sun salutation, relaxation pose
Poses to increase focus and balance (Appendix D): Tree pose, triangle pose, twisting triangle pose, revolving side angle, standing forward bend, cobra pose, bow pose, bridge pose, wheel pose, shoulderstand, plough pose

Diarrhea

What is Diarrhea?

Diarrhea is a condition when bowel movements become frequent and watery. Diarrhea may be accompanied by abdominal pain and cramping. Cancer-related diarrhea is often due to cancer treatments including chemotherapy, radiation therapy, bone marrow transplantation, and surgery, but can also be brought on by the cancer itself, infections, antibiotic therapy, and acquired food intolerance.

How is Diarrhea Treated by Conventional Medicine?

Because diarrhea can lead to dehydration, nutritional deficiencies, pain, and discomfort, preventative strategies and prompt intervention is important. Developing a plan to manage diarrhea depends on the cause of the diarrhea and may include diet changes that help firm the stool, discontinuing or reducing doses of laxative medications or stool softeners, or the use of opiate derived medications such as loperamide.

Integrative Approaches to Diarrhea

Nutrition is the cornerstone of an integrative approach to diarrhea. In most cases, we begin by counseling on dietary modifications. Supplements may be particularly helpful by providing adequate soluble fiber for those that are unable to eat foods high in soluble fiber. If the suggested changes in diet are not feasible, consider another therapy. The therapy that may be most beneficial will depend on your clinical condition and conventional medical plan.

Before adding any integrative therapy to your treatment plan, speak with your doctor about the benefits and risks. A summary of risks may be found in the Introduction along with detailed instructions for the application of and considerations for each of the indicated therapies.

Integrative Medicine in Action

Patient Story
Integrative Medicine Plan for Diarrhea:
Acupressure, Nutrition, and Reflexology.
Patient: Mary, a 75-year old woman diagnosed with pancreatic cancer experiencing severe diarrhea.
History and Complaint: Mary was experiencing frequent watery diarrhea after every meal and small snack. Mary had lost a significant amount of weight not only because of the diarrhea but because she refused to eat for fear she would feel uncomfortable and humiliated. She had lost 45 pounds since diagnosis and was experiencing extreme weakness, lethargy, and fatigue.
Treatment: Mary had to be reassured that although she felt humiliated by the diarrhea, it was a natural side effect of the chemotherapy and the cancer. Touch therapies such as reflexology and acupressure calmed her anxiety and helped balance her digestive system. Daily reflexology sessions administered by her daughter focused on the large and small intestines for balance, the spinal reflexes and solar plexus reflexes for relaxation, and the stomach reflex for increased appetite. Reflexology treatments helped her to feel well enough to eat small amounts of unsweetened rice, bananas, and avocados throughout the day. In between reflexology sessions, acupressure was applied to points Liv 3, PC 6, Ren 17, SP 6, SP 15, ST 25, and ST 37 for additional management of diarrhea and the emotional stress accompanying it.
Outcome: After a few weeks of reflexology, acupressure, and food changes, Mary felt a little stronger and was able to eat better. Not only did the reflexology and acupressure help her physically, but they were also helpful in calming her anxiety and regaining her strength.

Chinese Medicine/Acupressure

According to Chinese medicine, diarrhea refers to an increase in the frequency of bowel movements that are loose and contain undigested food or watery stool. In acute cases, the cause is generally seen as improper diet or invasion of dampness in the large intestine. In chronic cases, mental stress, certain medications, or prolonged illness is often the cause as these conditions will both deplete and inhibit the proper functioning of organs associated with digestion.

Acupressure
Most frequently used (Appendix A)
SP 15, ST 25, ST 37

Secondary points (Appendix A)

If accompanied by urgency, foul odor, and burning sensation around the anus, add: GB 34, LI 4, LI 11, SP 9

If worsened by emotional stress and possibly accompanied by belching and pain prior to bowel movement, add: Liv 3, PC 6, Ren 17, SP 6

If occurring in the early morning, with cold limbs and weak and sore low back and knees, add: DU 4, Kid 3, Ren 4, UB 23

Herbal Teas

A variety of teas may aid in the management of diarrhea. For the treatment of diarrhea, drink tea throughout the day. For prevention of diarrhea, drink the tea on a daily basis, once or twice per day. The most commonly used teas are slippery elm (*Ulmus rubra*), raspberry (*Rubus idaeus*), bilberry (*Vaccimium myrtillus*), and marshmallow root (*Althaea officinalis*). Raspberry and bilberry teas have the most appealing taste; however, slippery elm has a long history for helping ailments of the stomach and intestines. Simply select the tea that is most appealing to you. Avoid extremely hot or cold temperatures. Instructions for tea preparation may be found in Chapter 4.

- Bilberry. Seep 1 to 3 tsp of mashed herb in 8 ounces of warm water for 10 min, strain. Raspberry and bilberry can be combined for an additive effect.
- Blueberry. Add 3 tbsp of dried blueberries to 8 ounces of water and simmer for 5-10 minutes. Strain and drink at room temperature.
- Raspberry. Add 1 to 2 tsp to 8 ounces of water, seep for five minutes, strain.
- Slippery elm. Dilute 1 tsp of slippery elm in warm water, mix until herb is diluted in the water. Drink at room temperature.
- Marshmallow root. Add 3 tsp in 8 ounces of cold water, seep for 90 minutes, strain.

Homeopathy

For most patients suffering from diarrhea, a 30c potency is indicated (the more severe your diarrhea, the higher the potency). Begin with a few tablets as soon as you feel the urge of diarrhea, and then continue taking the tablets every 15 to 30 minutes until symptoms resolve. Do not exceed 6 doses per day. Discontinue supplementation when hard stools are passed. The most commonly suggested remedies are as follows:

- Aloe. Use for watery diarrhea accompanied by gas.

- Podophyllum. Use for diarrhea associated with a foul smell, watery stools, or for diarrhea that is painless or worse in the morning.

Massage

Choose this therapy especially when you are experiencing abdominal discomfort from diarrhea; avoid deep pressure. Information on the recommended massage technique may be found in Chapter 4.

Massage by a Caregiver

Self Massage

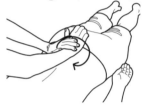 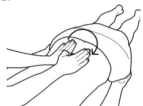 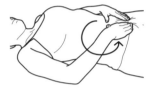

1 Massage in circular motions up and down the lower back on top of the sacrum (triangle shaped bone on the bottom of the spine) with the heel of your hand.

2 Massage with petrissage circular motions from the bottom of the sacrum up to and around the top of the buttocks.

1 Massage the lower belly with light petrissage technique.

2 Circle around the belly button keeping the palm of your hand flat against the skin. Move your hand in a counterclockwise direction.

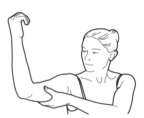 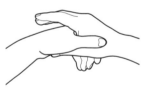 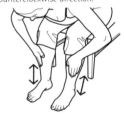

3 Massage the outside of the upper arm over the triceps with a petrissage grasping technique.

4 Pinch the web of the hand in between the forefinger and the thumb and apply light squeezing pressure.

5 Massage the outside of your shin bone on both legs with a petrissage up and down rubbing technique.

Nutrition

Diarrhea can be made better or worse by a variety of foods so it is important to pay attention to what you eat. Foods and drinks that worsen diarrhea are: high-sugar containing foods (cakes, cookies, candy, juice, soda); dairy (milk, ice cream, cheese); greasy foods (French fries, fried plantains, bacon, fried chicken); gas forming foods (beans, broccoli, Brussels sprouts, cauliflower, soda); foods high in insoluble fiber; caffeine. Not all of these foods will contribute to diarrhea in all people. Keep a list of the foods you eat to determine which foods make your diarrhea worse and avoid them. Extreme temperatures (food or drinks that are very hot or very cold) may also aggravate diarrhea.

Quick Dietary Tips

• Avoid foods that can make your diarrhea worse
• Be sure to replenish fluids. Drink plenty of water and avoid drinks high in sugar.

Chronic diarrhea will deplete your body of essential nutrients and electrolytes, so it is important to replenish what is being lost. Sport drinks will replenish electrolytes but have extra sugar, which can increase diarrhea. Bananas, avocados, apricots, coconut, and flavored soup broths are better choices as they can replenish electrolytes without added sugar. Avocados are an especially good source of potassium (975 mg of potassium per avocado). Sprinkle avocado with salt to provide additional sodium.

Food Remedies

• Coconut water and milk are excellent sources of iron, calcium, magnesium, phosphorous, and manganese and have the same electrolytic balance as your blood. For this reason coconut is often referred to as the "blood remedy." Coconut water is high in both potassium and sodium, whereas coconut milk is a good source of potassium but much lower in sodium. Drink coconut water or milk within one hour after an episode of diarrhea.
• Include prebiotic-containing foods to your daily meal plan. These foods are nutrition for the good bacteria found in your gut and help keep them nourished. Foods high in prebiotics are asparagus, bananas, beans, kefir, Jerusalem artichokes, chicory root, garlic, flax, leeks, onions, and whole wheat flour.
• Choose foods high in potassium (figs, yams, avocados, bananas, apricots).
• Choose foods high in soluble fiber. Soluble fiber intake should not exceed 10 grams per day. Food sources of soluble fiber are listed in Appendix F.
• In Chinese medicine, leeks and barley (high in soluble fiber) help manage diarrhea. Leeks are particularly good for chronic diarrhea, and barley is best suited for preventative purposes, especially if you are entering a phase of chemotherapy that is associated with severe diarrhea.
• Umeboshi plums or paste can be used in a variety of dishes. The paste is good as a side to cooked greens such as spinach, kale, or collard greens. Umeboshi vinegar can be substituted for red wine, balsamic, or apple vinegars in many dishes.

- Prepare a Congee and Date Soup for management of chronic diarrhea: Cook five seedless dates with one cup of congee (1 cup rice to 5 cups water). If you cannot find seedless dates, buy seeded dates and remove the seeds after cooking.

Reflexology

Choose this integrative therapy if your belly is tender. Use throughout the day or when you feel an acute urgency to pass a stool. Information on reflexology technique may be found in Chapter 4.

Foot Points
H: Sigmoid colon reflex
R: Adrenal reflexes
T: Ascending colon, descending colon, diaphragm, liver, transverse colon reflexes

Hand Points
R: Adrenal reflexes
T: Ascending colon, descending colon, diaphragm, liver, transverse colon reflexes

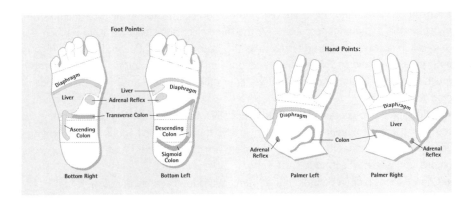

Supplements

Supplements may be especially helpful in managing chemotherapy- and radiation-induced diarrhea. The supplements are listed in order of preference, and may be combined for an additive effect.

- Blond psyllium is a form of soluble fiber. The dose is 9 grams taken two times per day. Blond psyllium must be taken with increased water. Take with calcium supplements (calcium carbonate, calcium phosphate) to make it more effective. If you are experiencing diarrhea related to tube feedings (tube inserted into the stomach), add blond psyllium to the formula, up to 30 grams per day as it may reduce diarrhea.

• **Probiotics.** Probiotics can be beneficial for the prevention and treatment of viral-induced infection and chemotherapy-induced diarrhea, particularly associated with 5-Fluorouracil or Topotecan. Probiotics may also be considered for radiation-induced diarrhea. Combining probiotics with fiber (see blond psyllium) may provide better management of diarrhea.

> Choosing a probiotic is difficult because there are so many different strains of pro-biotics and dosing is not simple. *Lactobacillus plantarum* is preferred for people undergoing cancer treatment. Doses of probiotics are measured by the number of living organisms (colony forming units (CFUs). Usually doses of 5 to 10 billion CFUs are recommended. Concentrated versions of probiotics contain up to 450 billion CFUs; however, these doses should be avoided during periods of severe immune suppression due to increased risk of developing an infection.

• Zinc. 10 to 40 mg of elemental zinc per day may enhance the benefits of other anti-diarrhea interventions, especially if you have diarrhea associated with malnutrition. Diarrhea can also be associated with zinc deficiency which can be monitored by blood tests.

Yoga

Deep breathing and relaxation can help relieve abdominal pain and spasms. Practice deep breathing and relaxation pose throughout the day.

Breathing (Appendix D): Alternate nostril breathing
Poses (Appendix D): Relaxation pose

Dry Mouth

What is Dry Mouth?

Xerostomia is the medical term for "dry mouth," a temporary or chronic condition of abnormal dryness of the mouth due to decreased secretions of saliva. Dry mouth occurs most often because of radiation therapy to the head and neck but may also develop from exposure to certain chemotherapeutic agents such as doxorubicin, surgery to the head and neck, or from infection. Dry mouth may lead to difficulty eating, sleeping, and speaking, and may be acute or chronic.

How is Dry Mouth Treated by Conventional Medicine?

Sensations of thick, sticky saliva and dryness of the mouth are best treated with frequent sips of water, mouth care after each meal and at bedtime, salt water rinses, fluoride gels or rinses to reduce tooth decay, dietary lubricating agents (olive oil, butter), or commercially prepared saliva substitutes. A diet of soft, moist foods may also help. For more severe, chronic dry mouth, the prescription medication, pilocarpine, may help increase saliva production in the mouth.

Integrative Approaches to Dry Mouth

Integrative strategies to treat dry mouth emphasize changes in diet along with touch therapies. The recommended dietary changes will help maintain calories during periods of dry mouth. Some of the recommended therapies are locally administered, that is they are administered right around the area of the mouth. In our practice, we frequently enlist the help of an acupuncturist to manage dry mouth, so you may consider consultation with a licensed acupuncturist. Between acupuncture visits, acupressure can provide sustained effects. Visual imagery may also provide relief from dry mouth by focusing your mind and allowing you to imagine moisture in your mouth.

Before adding any integrative therapy to your treatment plan, speak with your doctor about the benefits and risks. A summary of risks may be found in the Introduction along with detailed instructions for the application of and considerations for each of the indicated therapies.

Integrative Medicine in Action

Patient Story
Integrative Medicine Plan for Dry Mouth:
Acupressure, Massage, and Visual Imagery.
Patient: Brian, a 33-year old man undergoing radiation therapy for head and neck cancer presenting with dry mouth.
History and Complaint: After a series of radiation treatments, Brian started to lose the ability to produce saliva. Feeling frustrated, he lost interest in eating.
Treatment: Brian complemented his prescribed medications for dry mouth and weekly acupuncture sessions with acupressure and massage. Brian received acupressure from his wife on the points LI 3, LI 4, Ren 23, and ST 6 while sucking on a lemon candy. Following the acupressure session, his wife gently massaged the muscles in his face using a petrissage motion. Feeling relaxed, his wife then asked him to close his eyes and follow a ten minute visual imagery which guided him to relax his jaw, imagine saliva gathering in his mouth, and feel the juice of a lemon inside his mouth.
Outcome: Brian felt a gradual increase in moisture in his mouth through this integrative approach. During periods of dry mouth, he continued to practice the visual imagery to relieve his discomfort.

Chinese Medicine/Acupressure

In TCM theory, dry mouth and thick saliva indicate a lack of fluids or a thickening of fluids. Radiation therapy causes heat in a local area that can cause a drying up of fluids and/or impede the mechanism by which fluids would normally travel in order to provide lubrication. Treatment is typically centered on clearing heat and regulating the flow of qi to the mouth and throat.

Acupressure
Most frequently used (Appendix A)
LI 3, LI 4, Ren 23, ST 6
Secondary points (Appendix A)
If there is thick phlegm, add: Ren 9, Ren 12, ST 40
If accompanied by tightness in the chest, add: LU 1, PC 6, Ren 17
If accompanied by sores in the mouth, add: HT 8, ST 44
If there is feeling of a feverish sensation in the body, add: LI 11, LU 5, PC 5
Tip: It can be useful to suck on hard candy while applying acupressure to help stimulate the salivary glands.

Herbal Teas

The mild to strong bitter flavor of the following teas may provide some relief for dry mouth. Avoid the addition of sweeteners as this will decrease the benefit of the tea. Instructions for tea preparation may be found in Chapter 4.

• Green Tea (*Camellia sinensis*). Drink 2 to 3 cups of tea throughout the day. The tea can be prepared in a mild (1 to 2 tsp per 8 ounces) to strong (2 to 4 tsp per 8 ounces) flavor depending on your preference.
• Mild bitters. Yarrow (*Achillea millefolium*) 1/2 - 1 1/2 tsp to 8 ounces of boiling water, seep for 10 to 15 minutes, strain.
• Slippery elm (*Ulmus rubra*). (1 tsp per 8 ounces) or chamomile (*Matricaria recutita*) (2 to 4 tsp per 8 ounces) of boiling water, seep 5 to 10 minutes, strain. Add aloe vera juice (1 to 2 tbsp) to the tea.

Massage

Massage may help in stimulating the area around the glands that secrete saliva. You can use self massage as needed throughout the day. If you have lymphoma, do not massage directly over the lymph nodes (or "glands") in the neck. If you are unclear where these glands are located, ask a member of your medical team. Information on the recommended massage techniques may be found in Chapter 4.

Massage by a Caregiver

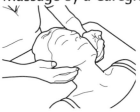 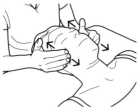 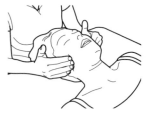

1 Massage the anterior digastric muscle where the front of the neck meets the jaw just under the angle. Use a cross ber friction technique by pressing up against the jaw bone.

2 Massage the masseter muscle on the cheeks of the face. Have the person clench their jaw if possible to cause the muscle to bulge out.

3 Have them relax the jaw and slightly open their mouth. Massage the muscle directly in front of the ear with a circular friction technique.

Self Massage

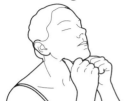 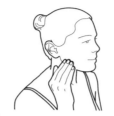 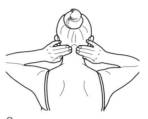

1 Lightly massage the muscles just under the where the neck meets the jaw (anterior digastric muscle) with a cross ber friction technique under the chin and jaw.

2 Massage the muscles of the cheeks one at a time. These are called the masseter muscles or the teeth clenching muscles. Apply circular motions over the muscle, then apply cross fiber friction again.

3 Massage the back of the neck where it meets the back of the head.

Nutrition

Dry mouth can be frustrating and may lead to lack of interest in food with subsequent effects on food intake weight loss. Drink plenty of liquids throughout the day; lemon water is a particularly good choice. Avoid caffeinated beverages (sodas, black teas, coffee, chocolate), alcohol, and high sugar foods as these will make your dry mouth worse. Choose tart and bitter flavors and foods that are moist and easy to swallow. Avoid dry foods such as crackers, bread, raw vegetables, and dried fruit. If you are having trouble maintaining your weight due to dry mouth, review the recommendations in the chapter on Loss of Appetite. Make sure to drink water or lemon water with every few bites of food.

Quick Dietary Tips

• Choose soft foods and calorie-rich liquids (smoothies, high-protein drinks)
• Emphasize high calorie soup, yogurt, and sauces
• Avoid foods that dry your mouth such as crackers, dried fruit, dry or thick solid foods (meat, poultry, largely cut pieces of fruit or vegetables, plain rice or pasta)

Food Remedies

• Add sweet or tart foods to increase the flow of saliva and make your mouth feel less dry. Add lemon slices or lemon juice to water or sodas. Warm lemon juice or lemonade may also help.
• Use flavorful oils to lubricate the mouth before meals. Examples include extra-virgin olive oil, flaxseed oil, and sesame oil.

- Prepare calorie-rich pureed soups such as butternut squash, lentil, pea, or cream of broccoli.
- Bitter lettuce (such as dandelion, endive, chicory) or vegetables can be cooked or eaten as a salad. Add a generous amount of citrus-based dressing (either lemon or orange) for extra calories and to maintain moisture in the salad.
- Eat thin, hot cereals such as cream of wheat, farina, or congee.
- Try melon, pineapple, or papaya fruit nectars (nectars are preferred over juice). Mix one cup of papaya or peach nectar with 1/2 cup seltzer or sparkling water.
- Experiment with umeboshi plums or paste.
- Use ice pops, sorbet, frozen yogurt, and flavored ice chips to help keep your mouth moist throughout the day. Choose citrus, tropical fruit, or green tea flavors.
- Choose yogurt with fresh tropical fruits such as pineapple or papaya. If you are losing weight, a full fat (whole milk) yogurt is a better choice.

Reflexology

Choose reflexology if you are unable to use the massage recommendations. Apply reflexology before eating. Information on reflexology technique may be found in Chapter 4.

Foot Points
F: Mouth points on the big toe, specifically the base of the nail of the great toe, all the other toes particularly around the distal joints or behind the nails

Hand Points
F: Mouth points on the thumb, specifically the base of the nail of the thumb and the distal joints and above on the dorsal side of the fingers

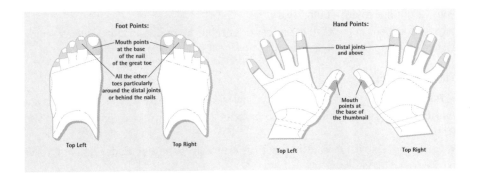

Visual Imagery

Sit with your back straight on a chair. Close your eyes and focus on your breath. Breathe in and out through the nose. Deep breath in, deep breath out. Take at least 7 to 10 seconds for each inhalation and each exhalation. Feel your body become more and more relaxed. *Focus on your breathing for at least 3 to 5 minutes.*

Now, bring your focus to the inside of your throat. Feel your throat start to moisten. Imagine you are drinking a cool glass of water. Feel that water moistening your throat. Feel that moistening rise up to the back of your mouth. Now imagine you are sucking on a lemon. Smell the lemon, taste the lemon, feel the lemon juice filling your mouth. Feel the salivary glands on the side of your mouth producing a moistening liquid. *Allow this feeling to be with your throat and your mouth for a several seconds.*

Slowly let the image go. Know that you can go back to this visualization every time you feel your mouth start to dry up. You can imagine you are sucking on a lemon anytime during your daily course of activities by taking just a moment to visualize and feel. Come back to awareness of the room you are in and the chair you are sitting on.

Slowly open your eyes.

Fatigue

What is Fatigue?

Fatigue is a common and often stressful condition experienced by many people undergoing cancer treatment. Acute fatigue is a sense of tiredness that can be resolved with rest while chronic fatigue, often called "cancer fatigue," is a persistent sense of ongoing exhaustion not relieved with rest.

Many factors may lead to fatigue including anemia, loss of appetite, shortness of breath, poor nutrition and inactivity, emotional distress, pain, and cancer treatment. Fatigue experienced during chemotherapy treatments is often worse in the days following treatment and then gradually subsides. Fatigue during radiation therapy generally increases as treatment progresses and does not resolve until after the radiation therapy is completed. Fatigue can also persist for many months upon completion of cancer therapy.

How is Fatigue Treated by Conventional Medicine?

Treatment of fatigue is most often geared towards addressing the symptoms of fatigue and providing emotional support. Treatments for fatigue include a thorough anemia evaluation, pain medication adjustments, exercise programs, and cognitive behavior therapy. For fatigue associated with anemia, dietary supplements may be helpful. Medications with potential benefits include psychostimulants (caffeine, methylphenidate, modafinil, dextroamphetamine). Epoetin alfa (Epogen® and Procrit®) and darbepoetin alfa (Aranesp®) are medications for the treatment of cancer-related anemia and may also help with symptoms of fatigue.

Integrative Approaches to Fatigue

Many different integrative therapies help manage fatigue. We advise most patients to choose one or more therapies that can be most easily woven into their lifestyles. For patients who enjoy athletics, yoga or exercise may be easy to incorporate into their current daily routines. Fatigue that becomes worse during or after a meal or snack may be relieved by dietary changes. Massage and acupressure can be particularly beneficial for fatigue associated with body weakness. Supplements may be appropriate for chronic fatigue or fatigue that persists upon completion of therapy.

Before adding any integrative therapy to your treatment plan, speak with your doctor about the benefits and risks. A summary of risks may be found in the Introduction along with detailed instructions for the application of and considerations for each of the indicated therapies.

Integrative Medicine in Action

Patient Story
Integrative Medicine Plan for Fatigue:
Nutrition, Supplements, and Yoga.
Patient: Richard, a 27-year old man with Hodgkin lymphoma experiencing chronic fatigue.
Chief Complaint: After four radiation treatments, Richard had grown so tired and weak he could barely make it out of bed. Although he slept most of the day, he never felt that he had enough energy to do even normal activities like eating. He could not concentrate, and his body, especially his arms and legs, felt extremely heavy.
Treatment: Richard did not want to take additional prescription medications because he was already taking three to five medications each day as part of his cancer treatment. Richard started by drinking one ounce of wheatgrass juice every day. He ate high-protein snacks, and small, low-glycemic meals, instead of large meals. He took four grams of L-carnitine per day. His oncologist recommended exercise, so Richard started practicing yoga every day and doing 30 minutes of mild cardiovascular exercise three times per week. Each afternoon he did three rounds of sun salutations to enhance his energy and a series of twisting postures for general circulation.
Outcome: Even after just the first week of incorporating these changes, Richard was able to get out of bed and had improved energy throughout the day.

Aromatherapy

Directly inhale the essential oils to obtain immediate relief from fatigue. The oils can also be applied to acupressure points. For physical fatigue, essential oils may be combined with a caregiver massage on your legs and feet with rosemary. Instructions for application of aromatherapy may be found in Chapter 4.

Compress: Black pepper, Fennel, Ginger. Apply the compress on the lower belly or lower back.
Diffusion/Direct Inhalation: Basil, Grapefruit, Peppermint.
Foot Bath/ Massage: Basil, Rosemary.
Special Applications
• Directly apply Ginger on acupressure points Ren 6 and ST 36 (Appendix A).
• Directly inhale Frankincense and Peppermint. Then, directly apply Peppermint at DU 20 (Appendix A) and massage along the base of the skull.

Chinese Medicine/Acupressure

Fatigue can affect the whole body or be localized (whole body muscle weakness compared to leg weakness). In TCM, fatigue can be caused by a deficiency of qi, which leads to the inability of qi to flow freely throughout the body. The goal of TCM is to stimulate the production of qi within the body and to regulate the flow of qi so it is able to reach all areas.

Acupressure

Most frequently used (Appendix A)
DU 20, Ren 6, Ren 12, ST 36

Secondary points (Appendix A)
If you are experiencing breathlessness, weak voice, and/or pale complexion, add: LU 9

If you experiencing poor appetite and/or loose stools, add: Ren 11, SP 3, ST 25

If you are experiencing muscle weakness in legs, add: ST 31, ST 36, ST 41

If you are experiencing muscle weakness in arms, add: LI 10, LI 15

If you are experiencing palpitations and/or spontaneous sweating, add: HT 5, LU 7, PC 6, Ren 17

If you are feeling cold, have cold limbs, and/or abdominal pain, add: Kid 7, SP 3, UB 20, UB 23

If accompanied by lack of motivation, soreness of the lower back and knees and/or frequent, pale urination, add: Kid 3, Kid 7, Ren 4, UB 23

If accompanied by palpitations, poor memory, and/or insomnia, add: HT 7, PC 6, Ren 17

If accompanied by slight numbness or tingling in limbs, bruising easily, and/or dry nails, skin or hair, add: Liv 8, Ren 4, UB 17, UB 18, UB 20

If accompanied by irritability, distended feeling under the ribcage or chest, nausea, and/or belching, add: GB 34, Liv 3, Liv 13, Liv 14, PC 6, SJ 6

If accompanied by headaches, dizziness, tinnitus, dry mouth and throat, and/or short temper, add: Kid 3, Liv 3, Liv 8, PC 7. For women add Ren 4 ; for men add HT 7

If accompanied by tremors, tics, numbness, dizziness, or paralysis, add: DU 16, GB 20, Liv 3, SI 3, UB 62

Herbal Teas

Choose any of the following teas and drink hot or warm. Avoid adding sweeteners. Instructions for tea preparation may be found in Chapter 4.

• Citrus. Choose from any citrus flavor such as orange, grapefruit, lemon, lime, or tangerine. Citrus teas are usually very palatable, and the strength of the tea will vary by individual preference. Use 1 to 4 tsp of any citrus tea in 8 ounces of hot water, seep for 5 to 10 minutes, strain.

- Peppermint (*Mentha piperita*). 1 to 2 tsp in 6 to 8 ounces of hot water, seep for 10 minutes, strain.
- Rosemary (*Rosmarinus officinalis*). 1 to 2 tsp in 6 to 8 ounces of boiling water, seep for 10 to15 minutes, strain.

Homeopathy

For acute onset fatigue that usually resolves within a few days, start with a dose of 30c. For chronic or severe fatigue, start with a lower potency (6c or 12c) and continue until you no longer have symptoms.

- **Carbo veg.** Fatigue associated with weakness, restlessness, sluggishness, and anxiety. Good for fatigue particularly associated with an illness.
- Gelsemium. Fatigue associated with both emotional and physical tiredness. Especially for those preferring quiet environments or experiencing feelings of fear.
- Phosphoricum acidum. Fatigue associated with indifference, apathy, or feelings of being overwhelmed.

Massage

Massage can be helpful for both acute and chronic fatigue. The massage techniques recommended for fatigue invigorate the circulation. You may want to consider incorporating aromatherapy into your massage to magnify the effect. Information on the recommended massage techniques may be found in Chapter 4.

Massage by a Caregiver

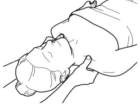 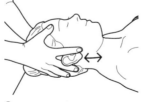 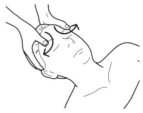

1 Have the person lie on their back. Using a petrissage grasping technique, massage the trapezius muscles on the neck/shoulder area. Apply some pressure so it becomes a slight pinching movement.

2 Spread your fore fingers and middle fingers to form a "V". Place them over and below the ears so the ear is in between them. Apply a brushing technique by sliding your fingers back and forth.

3 Next apply small circular pettrisage motions on the forehead and cheeks.

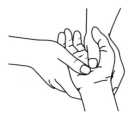

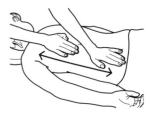

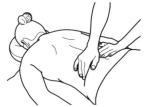

4 Use these same small circular pettrisage motions on each palm of hand.

5 Have them turn over onto their belly. Massage the entire back with long eflfeurage strokes.

6 Concentrate on the lower back using smaller petrissage strokes. Focus over the lower ribs down to the hip bones on the quadratus lumborum muscle.

Self Massage

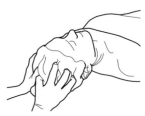

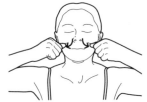

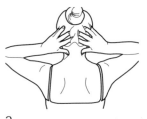

7 Finish by rubbing their head with a brushing motions as if you are washing their hair.

1 Slide the thumbs down each side of the nose with the nail side down.

2 Slide the thumbs under the cheek bones from the nose to the ears.

3 Use circular petrissage motion on the back of the head right above the neck with your four finger tips.

4 Brush your hair with your finger-tips from the forehead to the back of the head.

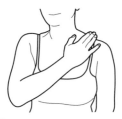

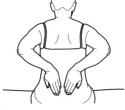

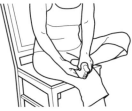

5 Using circular petrissage tech-nique, with the heel of your hand, massage the chest area above the breasts where the chest meets the front of the shoulder. One side at a time.

6 Massage the lower back over the lower ribs, the lower back itself, and over the buttocks with a petrissage brushing technique.

7 Using petrissage circular motion technique, massage the lower belly around the belly button (first in a clockwise motion and then counter-clockwise).

8 Massage the bottom of the feet with a petrissage grasping and small circular motion techniques. If you can't reach your feet, ask a caregiver to assist you with this step.

Nutrition

Poor nutrition may contribute to symptoms of fatigue. Small changes in your diet can help make fatigue more manageable. Pay attention to the quantity of food you are eating and the timing of your meals and snacks throughout the day. Most importantly, **avoid overeating**!

Quick Dietary Tips

- Emphasize foods that are low on the glycemic index
- Choose snacks rich in protein
- Eat small meals and avoid overeating

Eat small meals and high-protein snacks such as high-fiber crackers with cheese, nut butters, bean spreads, celery sticks with hummus or cream cheese, dried beans, and fresh or dried coconut. These foods will help you avoid elevations in your blood sugar that can promote feelings of tiredness. Choose foods that have a low glycemic index (Appendix E) as these foods prevent a lot of sugar from being released into your blood at one time.

Food Remedies

- Squeeze fresh lemon or lime on foods and in drinks. Lemon and lime are natural pick-me-ups.
- Add garlic to foods. The stronger the flavor, the more effective it is at improving fatigue.
- Brown rice balls are an easy "grab and go" snack. Prepare at home or buy at your local health food store. Cook one cup of brown rice until sticky. Roll a small handful of rice into a ball and coat by rolling or sprinkling with gomasio or a seaweed gomasio.
- Barley or wheat grass juice: Drink 1 to 2 ounces of juice per day (available in most health food stores). If fresh wheat grass juice is not available, you can juice fresh greens or use a ready-to-mix powder.

To prepare your own juice:

- o Kale (1 bunch)
- o Spinach (1 bunch)
- o Garlic to taste
- o Beets (especially if you have a low platelet count)
- o Ginger

Directions: Wash well and put through a juicing machine. For a slightly sweeter taste, add pure fresh apple juice.
- Use rosemary as a spice. Rosemary particularly helps with mental tiredness.

Reflexology

The technique and reflexology points focus on stimulating energy. Administer throughout the day as needed. Information on reflexology technique may be found in Chapter 4.

Foot Points
H: Pituitary reflexes
R: Adrenal reflexes
T: Diaphragm, solar plexus, spinal reflexes

Hand Points
F: Tips of fingers
H: Pituitary reflexes
T: Diaphragm, solar plexus reflexes; whole thumb, middle of palm

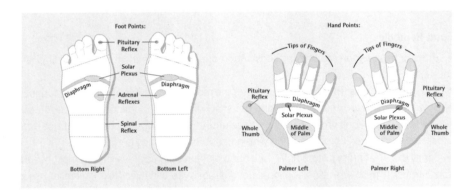

Supplements

Supplements may help with fatigue but caution with their use is warranted as there may be interactions with chemotherapy. Siberian ginseng and cordyceps should usually be avoided during chemotherapy. Siberian ginseng may only be considered after completion of cancer therapy. Cordyceps may also interfere with immunosuppressive agents such as cyclophosphamide and prednisone. L-carnitine may be an option during therapy as there is a low risk for an interaction with most chemotherapy drugs and radiation. Your doctor can help you choose the supplement that is best for your clinical condition.

• Cordyceps (*Cordyceps sinensis*). 2 to 3 grams per day.
• *L-carnitine.* 3 to 4 grams per day. Improvements in fatigue may be experienced within seven days of administration.

- Rhodiola (*Rhodiola rosea*). Doses suggested of 170 mg to 575 mg of the root extract. Start at the low end and increase as needed. Beneficial for stress-related fatigue.
- Siberian Ginseng *(Eleutherococcus senticosus)*. For mild fatigue, start with 2 grams per day. For persistent fatigue, you may increase the dose to 4 to 6 grams per day. Siberian ginseng can interact with many classes of drugs. Siberian ginseng should especially be avoided in individuals receiving chemotherapy for hormone sensitive cancers such as breast cancer, uterine cancer, ovarian cancer, and prostate.

Visual Imagery

Do not lie down for this visualization. Make sure you are sitting upright. Sit comfortably in a chair. The spine is upright and the feet are planted firmly on the floor. Take a deep breath. When you inhale, feel your belly pushing out. Take another deep inhalation so that your belly pushes out. When you exhale, make sure you are exhaling for at least 10 seconds. Do this several times.

Now that you are focused on your breath, tell yourself that every inhalation you take brings new, revitalizing energy to your body. Imagine that with every exhalation you are releasing old, stale, and tired energy. Inhale revitalizing energy, exhale old tired energy. Breathe in the energizing energy, breathe out the stale energy. Do this until you feel more revitalized. Keep telling yourself, "I breathe in new, revitalizing energy. I breathe out old, tired energy."

You should feel revitalized and energized after this visualization. Repeat as necessary.

Yoga

Yoga is a form of exercise that balances activity with rest and leaves you feeling refreshed and renewed. Yoga not only promotes strength but also improves circulation, builds energy, and helps maximize the quality of your sleep, thereby helping you manage your fatigue. If your fatigue is severe start by using the breathing techniques along with the first two yoga poses and relaxation pose. As your energy increases, continue on to complete the full yoga posture sequence (vinyasa).

Breathing (Appendix D): Ujjayi breath, kapalabhati, alternate nostril breathing
Poses (Appendix D): Sun salutation, twisting triangle pose, revolving side angle pose, straight leg seated spinal twist, cobra pose, bow pose, camel pose, bridge pose, wheel pose, supine twist, standing forward bend, relaxation pose

Headache

What is a Headache?

Headaches are usually experienced as pain above the eyes or ears, behind the head, or in the back of the upper neck. Headaches can occur frequently in patients with cancer and are generally divided into two main types. **Primary headaches** include migraines, cluster headaches, and tension or muscle contraction headaches, and **secondary headaches** are caused by another medical condition or underlying factor such as a brain tumor, infection, or medication.

Headaches may occur in patients with brain cancer or nasopharyngeal carcinoma or in patients who have cancer that has spread to the brain such as lung cancer, breast cancer, or melanoma. Headaches during cancer treatment may be caused by radiation therapy to large areas of the brain; biologic therapies such as interferons, monoclonal antibodies, or colony stimulating factors [filgrastim (Neupogen®), pegfilgrastim (Neulasta®), sargramostim (Leukine®)]; or chemotherapy agents including procarbazine, fluorouracil, and temozolomide. Conditions associated with cancer treatment including dehydration, anemia (low red blood cell count), infection, and high calcium levels in the blood may lead to headaches. Other medications used to manage side effects of chemotherapy such as ondansetron (Zofran®) may also be associated with headaches. Headaches can be made worse by stress, anxiety, and insomnia.

How are Headaches Treated by Conventional Medicine?

Headache symptoms differ in timing, frequency, duration, location, and severity. Depending on the symptoms, different medications may be prescribed to prevent or treat headaches. Medications include over-the-counter and prescription pain relievers (acetaminophen, ibuprofen, codeine), tricyclic antidepressants (amitriptyline hydrochloride), triptan medications (sumatriptan), corticosteroids (dexamethasone), or antibiotics. Red blood cell transfusions may also help with the headaches related to anemia.

Integrative Approaches to Headaches

Integrative therapies can be especially helpful in the management of headaches. In our practice, we begin with touch therapies. Touch therapies can provide instant relief, and repeated applications often have a sustained effect. Massage, reflexology, and acupressure may be combined or applied individually. Massage applied over the painful area can provide localized relief especially when combined with aromatherapy. Nutrition, supplements, teas, and yoga are better indicated for the prevention of chronic headaches.

If your headaches are related to diet, incorporate some of the suggested dietary strategies. Supplements may be beneficial if you are not experiencing relief from any of the manual therapies. Aromatherapy can also be added to a nutrition, herbal tea, or supplement regimen.

Before adding any integrative therapy to your treatment plan, speak with your doctor about the benefits and risks. A summary of risks may be found in the Introduction along with detailed instructions for the application of and considerations for each of the indicated therapies.

Integrative Medicine in Action

Patient Story
Integrative Medicine Plan for Headache:
Acupressure, Massage, and Reflexology.
Patient: Isaac, a 52-year old man with glioblastoma multiforme complaining of severe, debilitating headaches.
Chief Complaint: Isaac's headaches could not be fully relieved with the prescription medications. The headaches were less intense but still present. He often found it difficult to be around any stimulation such as lights, television, or computer games.
Treatment: After consulting with his doctor and an integrative medicine team, Isaac's wife decided to try massage, reflexology, and acupressure to help relieve his headaches. First she applied body lotion to his feet and legs to bring the pressure down and away from his head. She then massaged the tibialis anterior (muscles by the shin bone) and the gastrocnemius muscles (calf muscles) and applied thumbwalking to all the toes, particularly the big toe. Because her husband was anxious when experiencing pain, she also applied thumbwalking to the diaphragm, spinal, and neck shoulder reflexes. She applied acupressure to LI 4 and ST 44.
Outcome: Isaac reported that his headaches subsided following the massage, reflexology, and acupressure session, and he was able to come out of the dark.

Aromatherapy

Calming and uplifting essential oils can reduce tension headaches. For immediate relief, rub essential oils either on your temples or at the base of your neck. Be careful with the inhalation methods as too much inhalation of essential oils can cause a headache.

Aromatherapy is often combined with touch therapies. Instructions for application of aromatherapy may be found in Chapter 4.

Diffusion/Direct Inhalation/Massage: Grapefruit, Lavender, Peppermint, Roman chamomile.
Special Applications
• For congestion type headaches, directly inhale or diffuse Eucalyptus. Apply Eucalyptus on your palms, rub your hands together, and practice alternate nostril breathing (Appendix D). You can also put 2 to 5 drops of Eucalyptus on the base of the shower. Breathe deeply as the warm mist aerates your shower room.
• Directly apply Lavender or Peppermint to any of the foot reflexology points involving the toes listed in this section.
• For tension type headaches, directly massage a small amount of Tiger Balm (about 1/4 the size a small coin) or Lavender on your temples.
• Directly massage Peppermint on the trapezius muscle at the neck and shoulder area and over the muscles near the back of the skull.

Chinese Medicine/Acupressure

In TCM, headache can be caused by many factors. The cause of the headache is determined by the location of the pain, the quality (for example dull, throbbing), factors that make it better or worse (for example light, smells), and the circumstances present at the onset of the headache.

Acupressure
Most frequently used (Appendix A)
LI 4 (this is a common point for any type of headache and can have an immediate effect for alleviating pain)
Most frequently used according to location (Appendix A)
Occipital (back of the head): GB 20, SI 3
Frontal (forehead/front of head): DU 23, ST 8, ST 44
Temporal (side or sides of head): GB 8, GB 41, SJ 5, Tai Yang
Vertex (top of the head): DU 20, Kid 1, Liv 3
Secondary points (Appendix A)
With empty/hollow sensation or lingering mild/dull headache (may have dizziness), add: DU 20, GB 39, SP 6, ST 36
With heavy sensation, unclear thinking and dizziness, and/or nausea, add: DU 20, GB 34, PC 6, Ren 12, ST 8, ST 40
With fixed, stabbing, and/or throbbing pain, add: GB 43, Liv 3, SI 3, SP 10

Herbal Teas

Choose a flavorful tea and incorporate the tea into your daily routine while relaxing. Drink 1 to 3 cups of tea over the course of the day. Instructions for tea preparation may be found in Chapter 4.

- **For tension headaches:** Skullcap (*Scutellaria lateriflora*) and Wood betony (*Stachys officinalis*). 1 to 3 tsp to 6 to 8 ounces of hot water, seep for 10 minutes, strain.
- **For migraines:**
  o Feverfew (*Tanacetum parthenium*). 2 tsp in 6 to 8 ounces of hot water, seep for 15 minutes, strain.
  o Ginger (*Zingiber officinalis*). 1 tsp to 6 to 8 ounces of hot water, seep for 5 minutes, strain.
  o Lavender (*Lavandula spp*). 1 to 3 tsp to 6 to 8 ounces of hot water, seep for 10 minutes, strain.
  Combining several herbs often has a cumulative effect.
- **For headaches related to stress/anxiety:** The herbal teas found in this chapter can be combined with any of the teas found in the chapter entitled Anxiety & Stress. A combination of teas would be most beneficial.

Homeopathy

For acute headaches, select the remedy that best describes your headache and begin with a dose of 6x or 12x. Doses should be taken every 15 to 20 minutes until relief is experienced, up to 2 hours. For prevention, use a dose of 6x 1 to 2 times per day for a maximum of 4 to 6 weeks. Choose another integrative therapy for chronic and persistent headaches.

- **Belladonna.** Sudden onset, throbbing, high intensity pain, sinus pain, worsened by light, noise, and smell.
- **Bryonia.** For headaches characterized by stabbing pain related to stress, anxiety, anger, worsened by eye movement and touch.
- Gelsemium. For headaches characterized by dizziness, light-headedness, blurry vision, "heavy head," or associated with a burning sensation.
- Nux vomica. For "splitting headaches" due to loss of sleep, mental exhaustion, gastrointestinal upset, irritability. Headaches are often associated with excessive eating or drinking.

Massage

Massage by a caregiver is preferred if you are in too much pain to administer any therapy to yourself. Self massage can be very convenient when your headache is mild and you are comfortable enough to apply the strokes. Use throughout the day as needed. Information on the recommended massage technique may be found in Chapter 4.

Massage by a Caregiver

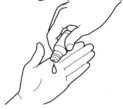

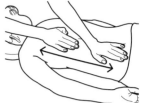

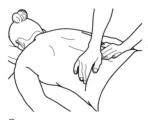

1 Put one drop of peppermint oil or a 1/4 the size of a small coin of Tiger Balm (refer to the aromatherapy section in this chapter) onto your hand. Add your base oil or body lotion/ cream. Lather your hands with the mixture.*

2 Have the person lie on their stomach. Massage with long ef- fleurage strokes to the paraspinal muscles along each side of the spine. Start at the upper back and move down.

3 Massage the lower back on the quadratus lumborum muscles (muscles above the hip bones) with circular and kneading petrissage motion.

*CAUTION: Avoid contact with eyes when using oil or balm.

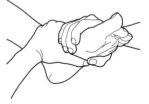

4 Using a light, grasping petrissage technique, massage the trapezius muscles. These muscles begin at the bottom of the skull and extend to the shoulders. Slide the palms of your hands in this direction (down the back of the neck and out to the shoulders) with small petrissage at palm strokes.

5 Have the person turn over on his or her back and finish by a general grasping and rubbing technique on each of the feet. You can then apply reexology to the bottoms of the feet.

Self Massage

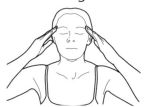 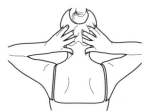 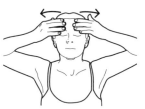

1 Put one drop of peppermint oil or a 1/4 the size of a small coin of Tiger Balm (refer to the aromatherapy section in this chapter) on your fingers, rub them together and, in a circular petrissage motion, lightly apply pressure to each temple with your fingertips.*

*CAUTION: Avoid contact with eyes when using oil or balm.

2 With your fingertips, apply a slightly deeper pressure on the back of your neck right under the skull or occiput region. Use a circular petrissage motion.

3 Put the palm side of your fingers flat against your forehead. The tips of the fingers on each hand should be touching one another. Slide them away from each other moving in an outward direction while keeping them flat against the forehead the whole time. This technique uses small petrissage strokes. Repeat 3 – 4 times.

Nutrition

Dietary changes may be helpful for primary headaches, such as migraines, especially if they are more chronic in nature. According to TCM, fatty foods (pork, fried foods), greasy foods, dishes prepared with heavy sauces, and ice cream should be avoided for all types of headaches. Clinical studies have found that a low fat diet (20 grams of fat per day) may help to decrease the incidence and severity of chronic migraines.

Caffeine intake may be related to headaches; however, rapid discontinuation of caffeine may also trigger headaches. Complete elimination of caffeine may not be necessary so a gradual reduction in intake is recommended.

Some headaches are related to food allergies and may be acquired during or after treatment for cancer. Foods that can trigger headaches are often highly individualized. Work with a nutritionist or registered dietician to help identify the offending foods. A thorough review of the timing and patterns of headaches in relation to food intake will help you identify possible dietary triggers. If indicated, an elimination strategy can be developed.

Reflexology

Reflexology is helpful because it brings the focus away from the pain of the head and onto the feet and hands. Information on reflexology technique may be found in Chapter 4.

Foot Points
F: All the toes, particularly from the distal joint to the tips, whole great toe
T: Diaphragm, spinal reflexes; neck/shoulder line

Hand Points
T: Diaphragm, spinal, whole thumb reflexes; neck/shoulder line

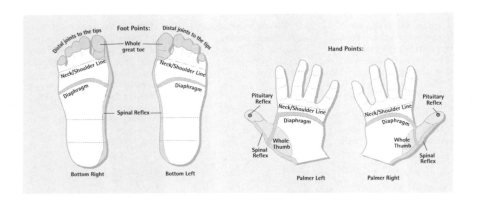

Supplements

Supplements may be considered for the prevention of headaches. If do you not experience relief, consider adding another supplement or combine supplements with another integrative therapy. Your doctor can help you choose a supplement that may be indicated to your clinical condition.

Prevention of Migraine Headaches
- **Butterbur (*Petasites hybridus*).** 75 mg 2 times per day for adults; 100 to 150 mg once per day for children 10 to 12 years old; and 50 to 75mg once per day for children ages 8 to 9 years.
- **Feverfew (*Tanacetum parthenium*).** 50 to 100 mg, standardized to 0.25 to 0.5 mg parthenolide, 2 times per day. This herb is especially helpful for frequent migraine attacks. A combination of feverfew, riboflavin, and magnesium may provide added benefit.
- **Magnesium.** 600 mg 3 times per day of magnesium citrate, maximum duration 3 months; 300 mg trimagnesium dicitrate, 2 times per day, maximum duration 3 months. For children, 9 mg per kilogram in 3 divided doses, maximum duration 4 months. Different forms of magnesium are available. Both high-dose magnesium citrate or trimagnesium in divided doses may reduce the frequency and severity of migraine headaches. Do not take

high-dose magnesium in a single dose. Be aware that high-dose magnesium may cause diarrhea, so increase your dose gradually, and do not use if you are experiencing chronic diarrhea.
- Riboflavin (B2). 400 mg per day.

Visual Imagery

Get comfortable. Take several deep breaths to relax your body and calm your mind. Feel the deep breaths all the way to your belly. Make sure you inhale through your nose and exhale out of your mouth. Do this for several minutes.

Now, focus your energy on the bottom of your feet. Feel all of the tension in your head drop down through your body into the bottom of the feet. Hold this visualization for several minutes. Now visualize all the dropped energy in your feet leave into the floor. Imagine a trap door opening at the bottom of your feet and the headache and pain falling through the door and into the floor. It continues to move down into the earth. See this energy continually moving from the head, through the body, into the feet, through the feet, and into the earth.

Repeat this visualization until you experience relief.

Yoga

By relaxing the mind and body, yoga may be useful for the prevention of headaches. Yoga may also provide relief at the early onset of a headache. Begin your yoga practice by relieving tension in your neck. To do so, practice some basic neck stretches, gently moving your head from side to side in preparation for your breathing exercises. Continue to relax into the suggested yoga poses by using the recommended supportive modifications described in the Appendix. Consider adopting a consistent yoga practice if you develop frequent headaches.

Breathing (Appendix D): Ujjayi breath, alternate nostril breathing
Poses (Appendix D): Legs up relaxation pose, relaxation pose

Hot Flashes

What are Hot Flashes?

Hot flashes, associated with natural or treatment-related menopause or with treatment for breast cancer or prostate cancer, are a sudden onset of body warmth, flushing, and sweating that lasts between a few seconds to minutes. Hot flashes that occur at night may be referred to as night sweats and are often more intense than hot flashes during the day. Night sweats can interfere with sleep and may lead to irritability, fatigue, memory loss, nervousness, depression, and anxiety.

How are Hot Flashes treated by Conventional Medicine?

Hot flashes associated with natural or treatment-related menopause can be controlled with estrogen replacement therapy, but its use is contraindicated in a number of medical conditions and hormone-sensitive cancers including breast and prostate cancer, as replacement therapy may increase risk of cancer recurrence. Other non-estrogen drugs, including megestrol or the antidepressant venlafaxine, may be prescribed in these cases. Doctors may also suggest wearing loose-fitting cotton clothing and the use of fans to keep the body temperature down.

Integrative Approaches to Hot Flashes

Most often integrative medicine should be tailored to manage the intensity and frequency of hot flashes. For mild hot flashes, consider aromatherapy, as it is especially good for cooling down the body during and after a hot flash. For severe hot flashes, consider visiting a licensed acupuncturist for individualized treatment. Acupressure can then further support your sessions of acupuncture. Nutrition can help for both mild and severe hot flashes and should be followed daily. Visual imagery and yoga can support any integrative therapy.

Many supplements such as red clover, dongquai, and chaste tree berry are believed to be helpful for hot flashes because they contain plant phytoestrogens, compounds that exert estrogen-like properties in the human body. Phytoestrogens can be obtained through supplements or food (Refer to the nutrition section in this chapter). The safety of phytoestrogens, especially from supplements, in patients with hormone-sensitive cancer is not completely understood, and especially in patients advised to avoid estrogen supplementation. It is not clear if supplements containing phytoestrogens can increase the risk of cancer recurrence or decrease the effectiveness of cancer therapy in individuals with breast or other hormone-sensitive cancers. **In this chapter, we do not recommend supplements containing phytoestrogens.** It is important to speak with your doctor before beginning any supplement or diet high in phytoestrogens.

Before adding any integrative therapy to your treatment plan, speak with your doctor about the benefits and risks. A summary of risks may be found in the Introduction along with detailed instructions for the application of and considerations for each of the indicated therapies.

Integrative Medicine in Action

Patient Story
Integrative Medicine Plan for Hot Flashes:
Acupuncture, Aromatherapy, and Nutrition.
Patient: Elizabeth, a 44-year old woman with estrogen receptor positive breast cancer experiencing hot flashes while receiving Tamoxifen therapy.
Chief Complaint: Elizabeth felt a surge of heat in her body, starting internally and then emerging in her face, neck, and chest. Elizabeth would then break out with profuse sweats which then made her feel a cool clamminess all over her body. The hot flashes, which she experienced every two hours, started in the day and continued throughout the night.
Treatment: Elizabeth sought assistance from a licensed acupuncturist. She received acupuncture and was educated on a weekly routine of self acupressure using points Kid 3, LI 11, Liv 3, and SP 6. Elizabeth carried peppermint oil and when she experienced a hot flash she would apply it to the back of her head and the bottom of her feet (at Kid 1). Elizabeth also followed the nutrition guidelines that included reducing saturated fat intake, increasing consumption of whole grains and striving for 4 to 6 fruits and vegetables each day.
Outcome: The hot flashes continued, but with less intensity and frequency. Elizabeth reported to her oncologist that the integrative plan was beneficial for managing her hot flashes.

Aromatherapy

Essential oils that are part of the mint family can be extremely cooling. For immediate relief of a hot flash, massage an essential oil on the back of the neck. Consider a cooling foot bath before going to sleep. Instructions for application of aromatherapy may be found in Chapter 4.

Bath/Direct Application/Direct Inhalation/Foot Bath: Peppermint, Spearmint, Wintergreen. Direct application should focus on the wrists, back of the neck, and feet.
Special Applications
- Directly apply Peppermint on acupressure point Kid 1 (Appendix A).

Chinese Medicine/Acupressure

In TCM the temperature regulation is related to the balance of yin (cold) and yang (heat) within our bodies. When we encounter certain circumstances that interfere with this balance, such as chemotherapy, we can experience our body temperature at certain extremes. One of these extremes is a rush or flash of heat such as hot flashes.

One aspect of the relationship between yin and yang is the ability of each to balance the other within our body. For example, when the yin of our bodies is depleted, it may be unable to "anchor" yang. Since it is the nature of heat to rise, this can result in an upward rush of yang, as in hot flashes. In Chinese medicine, we seek to supplement yin and anchor yang to reduce the frequency and severity of hot flashes.

Most frequently used (Appendix A)
GB 20, Kid 3, LI 11, Liv 3, Ren 4, SP 6
Secondary points (Appendix A)
Kid 1, Kid 6, LI 4, Liv 2, Liv 8, LU 7, PC 7, SP 4
With cold sensation and fatigue immediately following hot flash, add: Kid 7, UB 23
If accompanied by heart palpitations, add: HT 6, HT 8, LU 10, UB 15

Homeopathy

In homeopathic medicine, Belladonna is the most common recommendation for hot flashes. Begin with belladonna at a dose of 30x 3 times per day for 5 days. If no relief is obtained, consider another remedy. With the help of a homeopath, you may also want to consider combination remedies.

- **Belladonna.** Hot flashes with a sudden onset, intense heat, reddened face, and sweating.
- Sanguinaria. Hot flashes associated with headaches.
- Sepia. Hot flashes associated with movement. Mood swings, vaginal dryness, and decreased libido are often present.

Nutrition

Dietary change is a strategy that can help in the management of hot flashes. Changes in diet can include the addition of specific dietary nutrients (specific vitamins, soy, lignans) or the adoption of a comprehensive dietary plan such as a low fat diet.

The addition of soy to the diet is one of the most popular dietary changes for the management of hot flashes. The interest in soy has been driven by scientific observations reporting that women whose diets are high in soy have a decreased incidence of breast cancer and menopausal symptoms. Soy is a rich source of protein, vitamins, minerals, and isoflavones. Isoflavones are phytoestrogens or plant-based estrogens that naturally occur in soy. Since isoflavones can act like estrogen in the human body, the relationship between soy and menopausal symptoms has primarily been attributed to the isoflavones. Foods high in isoflavones are soy milk, tofu, tempeh, and miso. These foods provide approximately 40 mg of isoflavones per serving.

The effect of soy on menopausal symptoms has been evaluated in multiple clinical studies. In these studies, isoflavones were administered to participants in the form of concentrated powders at doses ranging from 35 to 150 mg per day. Results from these clinical studies suggest that soy is unlikely to help with the management of hot flashes or night sweats. However, in some individuals who are able to break down soy products into specific compounds, soy intake may be beneficial. The breakdown and absorption of these compounds is related to the individual's genetic make-up and gut microflora. Speak with your doctor or nutritionist to determine if soy might be right for you.

Lignans are another class of phytoestrogens that have also been found to help manage symptoms of menopause. Flaxseed provides the greatest amount of lignans but lignans can also be found in whole grains (multi-grain or rye bread, muesli, whole grain rice), vegetables (broccoli, Brussels sprouts, cabbage, kale), fruits (apricots, peaches, strawberries) and teas (Black tea, English blend, Earl Grey, green tea). Lignans appear to be safe among women with breast cancer. Clinical studies in humans have found that incorporating 40 grams of lignans every day into your diet may decrease menopausal symptoms.

Comprehensive dietary change may also help with symptoms of menopause. Following a diet that is composed of 20% of calories from fat (about 35 to 50 grams of fat per day), at least five servings of fruits and vegetables per day (Appendix G), and six servings of whole grains per day may alleviate hot flashes and night sweats. Adoption of this diet may be particularly beneficial for women experiencing hot flashes throughout the day and night sweats.

Many professionals advocate avoidance of hot, spicy foods, alcohol, and caffeine as these can make hot flashes worse.

Supplements

Clinical trials support the effectiveness of vitamin E in the management of hot flashes. Discontinue if relief if not obtained after a 2 to 3 months.

- Vitamin E. 400 IU 2 times per day.

Visual Imagery

As you feel a hot flash coming on, close your eyes, making sure you are in a safe area to do so and immediately focus on your feet. Imagine your feet are soaking in a cold river. Imagine you feel the crisp cold water running over the tops and bottom of your feet. Feel your body immediately start to cool off. Keep the focus on your feet.

Once the cool river water cools down your feet, imagine the heat that is overtaking your body rush downwards. Feel the heat leaving your face and head move downwards. Feel the heat in your chest, back, arms and belly move downwards. Feel the heat leaving your pelvis and legs move down to your feet.

Imagine an opening in the center of the bottom of your feet, like a portal. Imagine the heat pouring out of this opening into the cool river. Imagine the river immediately cooling off the heat that is leaving your body in a downward motion into the water.

Now imagine your entire body is cool. Tell yourself that your body will remain cool. Remind yourself that every time you feel a hot flash coming, the heat will move down and out of your feet into a cooling river of moving water carrying the heat away from you.

Tell yourself, "My body remains cool as the heat travels down to, and through my feet into cooling water."

Repeat as needed, up to several times a day as necessary.

Yoga

The suggested sequence of yoga postures lessens the intensity of the hot flash or sweat by lowering your heart rate and calming your nervous system.

Breathing (Appendix D): Ujjayi breath, alternate nostril breathing
Poses (Appendix D): Shoulderstand, plough pose, legs up relaxation pose, relaxation pose

Immune Suppression

What is Immune Suppression?

The immune system is responsible for fighting harmful organisms that cause infection. Immune suppression occurs when the cells of our immune system do not function efficiently and are not able to fight infection-causing organisms. More specifically, immune suppression occurs when there are low numbers of white blood cells, which can lead to an increased risk of infection. Low numbers of one type of white blood cell, the neutrophil, can lead to very serious bacterial or fungal infections.

Immune suppression occurs as a side effect of many chemotherapy drugs or following the administration of certain chemotherapy drugs or radiation therapy in preparation for bone marrow transplantation. Certain cancers such as leukemia also cause immune suppression.

How is Immune Suppression Treated by Conventional Medicine?

Depending on the anticipated severity of immune suppression, various preventative behavioral measures will be recommended. As a first line of defense, oncologists will emphasize good hand washing practices, minimizing exposure to others who are not feeling well, peeling and washing all fruits and vegetables, and eating meat well-done. As immune suppression can be more severe before, during, and after bone marrow transplantation, additional measures may be recommended; these can include wearing a mask, isolation from others, minimizing public transport and exposure to plants and animals, and adopting a low bacterial diet (the neutropenic diet).

In order to prevent or reduce the risk of infection during periods of immune suppression, hematopoietic growth factors [such as filgrastim (Neupogen®), pegfilgrastim (Neulasta®), sargramostim (Leukine®)], prophylactic antibiotics, or prophylactic antifungal medications may be used. If signs of infection are present, aggressive treatment with antibiotic, antifungal, or antiviral therapy, often requiring hospitalization, may be initiated prior to identification of the infectious organism.

Integrative Approaches to Immune Suppression

Integrative approaches overlap with conventional strategies in that the goal is to reduce the risk of an infection and enhance the immune system. Integrative nutrition recommendations emphasize food safety and foods high in phytonutrients, whereas supplements aim to support the immune system and retain the healthy flora in the gut to decrease the risk of bacteria moving into the bloodstream. Massage is the preferred touch therapy to support the immune and lymphatic system. Acupressure, aromatherapy, reflexology, and yoga can be used as an adjunct to any of the aforementioned therapies.

If you are experiencing other side effects that may increase your risk of an infection such as mouth sores, refer to the indicated chapter for additional strategies.

Before adding any integrative therapy to your treatment plan, speak with your doctor about the benefits and risks. A summary of risks may be found in the Introduction along with detailed instructions for the application of and considerations for each of the indicated therapies.

Integrative Medicine in Action

Patient Story
Integrative Medicine Plan for Immune Suppression:
Massage, Nutrition, and Supplements.
Patient: Lorna, a 46-year old woman with immune suppression following therapy for Acute Myeloid Leukemia.
Chief Complaint: After initiation of chemotherapy, Lorna's white blood cell count was low, but she had no signs of infection. She felt weak and was worried about supporting her body's immune response even with the administration of prophylactic antibiotics.
Treatment: Concerned about Lorna's overall weakness, Lorna's sister decided to give her frequent massages using the Manual Lymphatic Drainage technique after learning about its benefits. Her sister prepared a vegetable juice, and added whey protein to her yogurt along with a high fiber cereal every day for breakfast. She packed her diet with immune supporting foods like dried mushrooms, and spices such as turmeric, garlic, and onions.
Outcome: Lorna's white blood cell count gradually normalized, and she did not develop any life threatening complications.

Aromatherapy

Historically, the diffusion of essential oils like Frankincense and Myrrh has been used to increase immune function and to prevent infection. Essential oils may be diffused daily or as needed. Instructions for application of aromatherapy may be found in Chapter 4.

Bath: Rose
Diffusion/Direct Inhalation: Frankincense, Myrrh, Orange, Rose

Direct Application/Massage: Oregano, Thyme. Massage and direct application should focus on the feet.

Special Applications

• Directly apply Orange on acupressure point ST 36 (Appendix A).

Chinese Medicine/Acupressure

According to Chinese medicine, immune suppression refers to a deficiency of one or more of the vital substances in the body. Although applying acupressure to the specific points listed below can be helpful to boost the immune system, Chinese medicine should be used along with the recommendations made within the nutrition and supplements sections of this chapter.

Acupressure

Most frequently used (Appendix A)

Kid 3, Ren 4, SP 6, ST 36, UB 43

Massage

The massage technique suggested for immune suppression is lymphatic drainage. The goal for the caregiver is to massage the entire body to move the lymphatic system. Choose massage therapy alone or in combination with any other integrative therapies. Information on the recommended massage technique may be found in Chapter 4.

Massage by a Caregiver

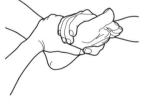 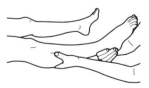 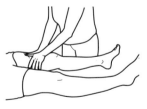

1 Start with one of the ankles by using a petrissage grasping technique.

2 With a repeated pumping motion (grasp, let go, grasp, let go, grasp, let go), work your way up from the ankle to the knee.

3 Continue with the grasping technique with both hands from the knee to the top of the thigh on the quadricep muscles.

4 Repeat on the other leg.

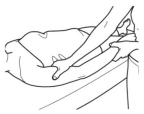

5 Starting at awrist, repeat the same process from the wrist to the shoulder.

6 Repeat on other arm.

Self Massage

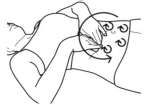
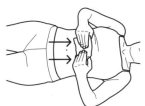
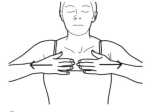

1 Massage the belly, first in clockwise circles around the belly button, then in counterclockwise circles.

2 Using your hands, a loofah, or washcloth, massage upward towards diaphragm with a sweeping petrissage motion.

3 Place the tops of your fingers or fingertips on your breast bone (in between the breasts on the sternum). Use the scraping petrissage technique and pull your fingers in an outward motion moving toward the sides of your body. Do this 3-4 times.

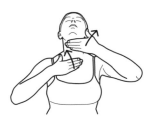
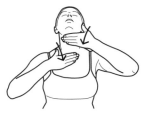

4 Next, apply the gentle sweeping technique in an upward direction on your neck moving towards the bottom of your chin.

5 Moving down from under the chin to the collar bones, repeat the sweeping petrissage technique. Do this 3-4 times.

Nutrition

Nutrition therapy is important in reducing your risk of infection when your white blood cell count is low. Focus on the immune-supportive foods by including them every day in your diet. The foods listed in this chapter have historically been used to support the immune system or are listed to support the gut and prevent harmful bacteria from making your gut their home.

At times during treatment when infection risk is especially high, your doctor might recommend a neutropenic diet, especially if your therapy includes a stem cell transplant. The details of this diet will vary depending on your doctor or the hospital where you are receiving treatment. In general, the diet strictly

• Follow food safety guidelines throughout your treatment
• Choose an immune-boosting food at least 3 times per day
• Diversify your diet so that you get exposed to a variety of nutrients that support your immune system

limits the type of foods you can eat such as fresh fruits and vegetables, salads, raw fish, and food from street vendors. This diet can be frustrating and limited in the foods that you can eat. Speak with your doctor to determine if this diet is absolutely necessary for you.

When you are immunosupressed or neutropenic, it is **essential** to follow food safety guidelines to help prevent any food-borne illness, especially as food borne illnesses are common, with nearly 1 in 4 adults in the United States experiencing an infection. General food safety recommendations are listed below. Additional information may be found at the Food and Drug Administration website (http://www.foodsafety.gov/).

• Wash all raw fruits and vegetables well. If the food cannot be washed well (as with raspberries), avoid it. Scrub rough surfaces, like the skin of melons, prior to cutting.
• Carefully wash your hands and food preparation surfaces (knives, cutting boards) before and after preparing food, especially after handling raw meat.
• Thaw meat in the refrigerator, not on the kitchen counter.
• Be sure to cook meat and eggs thoroughly.
• Avoid raw shellfish and fish and use only pasteurized or processed ciders and juices and pasteurized milk and cheese.
• Avoid salad bars and buffet-style restaurants.
• Do not share eating utensils or eat off of another person's plate.

Food Remedies

• Choose immune supporting foods: berries, cruciferous vegetables (kale, broccoli, Brussels sprouts, cauliflower), nuts (hazelnuts, cashews, pistachios), and complex carbohydrates (100% whole wheat bread, whole grain pasta or rice, vegetables, and fruits). For raspberries or blackberries, choose frozen over fresh to avoid possible bacterial contamination on the surface of the berry. Cruciferous vegetables should only be eaten cooked; especially during the periods of neutropenia.

• Start the day right. Change your breakfast cereal to a high-fiber cereal. If cereal is not appealing, try yogurt mixed with frozen berries. Add a small amount of agave nectar for flavoring. This is especially good if you are taking antibiotics for a long period of time.

• Juice. Green juices are recommended to support the immune system. You can use ready-to-mix green juice powders for ease of preparation. There are numerous brands on the market, so choose one that is made from primarily fruits and vegetables and does not have a lot of added foods or nutrients. You can add 100% pure apple juice or any other favorite juice for flavoring, if needed.

You can also purchase fresh vegetables and herbs and prepare them in a juice machine however you must wash them well and use within one day of purchase. Mix bunches of cabbage, celery, garlic, kale, parsley, red beets, and vegetable sprouts.

• Make an immune packed smoothie. Combine in a blender:

  o 1/2 to 1 banana (use more banana for a thicker consistency)
  o 1/2 cup organic yogurt made with whole or low fat milk
  o 1/2 to 1 cup of any milk-type product (dairy, soy, or rice milk)
  o 1 cup frozen berries
  o 2 to 4 tablespoons flax meal (depending on your preferred flavor)
  o 1/4 to 1/2 cup whey protein powder

• Incorporate sea vegetables into soups or salad. Arame and wakame are mild tasting sea vegetables.

• Eat one food item high in omega-3 fatty acids each day. Flax meal, fortified omega-3 eggs or cereals, and fish (canned or fresh sardines, Atlantic mackerel, Atlantic herring, Chinook salmon, Atlantic salmon, anchovy, lake trout, bluefish).

• Experiment with miso soup. Be generous with adding other immune-enhancing vegetables in the soup including mushrooms and seaweed.

• Choose from any of the listed mushroom varieties, Reishi, Maitaki, and Shitaki. Other varieties of mushrooms do not have the same nutritional value as those listed. Add these to any dish. Prepare only cooked mushrooms during periods of immune suppression.

• Be generous with spices. Turmeric, curry, cumin, coriander, garlic, onions, and cayenne pepper all support the immune system. Historically many of these herbs have been used to preserve foods to reduce the transmission of food-borne infections in hot climates.

• Experiment with prebiotic-containing foods to your daily meal plan. These foods are nutrition for the good bacteria found in your gut and help keep them nourished. Foods high in prebiotics are asparagus, bananas, beans, kefir, Jerusalem artichokes, chicory root, garlic, flax, leeks, onions, and whole wheat flour.

Reflexology

Reflexology can be applied along with acupressure or massage. Reflexology can be applied once a day or as needed. Information on reflexology technique can be found in Chapter 4.

Foot Points
F: Lymphatic drainage points "ditches"
H: Thymus reflexes
R: Adrenal reflexes

Hand Points
F: Lymphatic drainage points

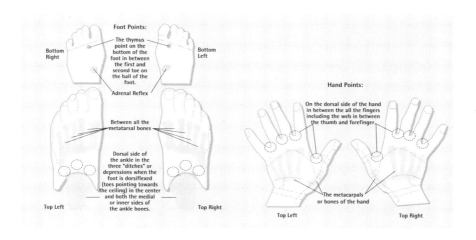

Supplements

In herbal medicine, supplements are recommended to support the immune system. Often, herbalists will suggest phytonutrients, compounds naturally found in foods, in a concentrated capsule or tablet form. Herbs that have historically been prescribed as "immune boosters" (e.g. goldenseal, panax ginseng) are typically suggested. **The safety of "immune boosters" is not known especially in the setting of stem cell transplant or immune-derived malignancies such as leukemia or lymphoma. Discuss supplementation with your doctor.**

- Mushroom mixtures. Mixtures of extracts of mushrooms may be found in most health food stores and are frequently recommended for patients undergoing treatment for cancer. Extracts of mushrooms may be a better choice if you do not prefer the flavor of mushrooms. Dosing will vary depending on the product. A qualified health professional will be able to provide guidance.
- Probiotics. Probiotics help reinforce the gut barrier thereby decreasing the risk of bacteria moving from the gut into the blood stream. Probiotics can be used during periods of high risk for infection or in patients who are severely immunocompromised. Refer to the chapter on diarrhea for species, dosing guidelines, and cautions.
- Shark liver oil or its active ingredient squalene. Although it is often taken as a cancer treatment, it has not yet been proven effective. Shark liver oil may function better as a support for the immune system. 50 mg 3 times per day is prescribed.
- Whey protein. Mix 30 to 50 grams of whey protein (usually 1 to 2 scoops, depending on the product) into a shake or any food product once daily.

Visual Imagery

Sit comfortably in a chair. Keep both feet planted on the ground. Make sure your spine is upright. Close your eyes. Take three deep breaths. Now imagine that your whole body is relaxed and receptive. Start at the top of your head. Imagine your face and head relaxing. Feel the muscles in your face let go of their tension. Feel your jaw opening. Feel the breath bringing more space into your mouth and throat as you relax. Now imagine this breath is opening and relaxing your throat. Now the relaxation goes across your chest and down into your arms. Now feel your belly relax. Your belly gets bigger with the breaths and the relaxation. Feel the tension leave your back and pelvis area. Now feel your legs letting go. Feel the tension in your knees, ankles, and feet start to dissipate.

Now that you are relaxed, with your mind's eye, imagine you can see inside your body. Visualize what every cell would look like. If you can, see every cell in your body as a spark of golden yellow light. See your cells alive and healthy. Tell your cells that they are alive and healthy. Tell yourself that as your cells vibrate with this vivid golden yellow light, like sparkling stars in a night sky, your immune system gets stronger. Visualize the healthy cells taking over. See all the unhealthy cells shrink, wither, and disappear. Healthy cells are vibrating, unhealthy cells are disappearing. Keep this visualization for as long as needed.

Now tell yourself that as your cells get healthier with this golden yellow light, your immune system gets stronger and stronger. Stay with it until you can see your whole body from the inside vibrating with healthy golden yellow cells.

Repeat daily.

Yoga

Daily yoga practice will help your body maintain strength during periods of immunosuppression. Chest opening poses and inversions stimulate the flow of lymph and immune cells throughout the body. Begin with the breathing and sun salutation. Add additional poses as you become confident with the vinyasa.

Breathing (Appendix D): Ujjayi breath, kapalabhati, alternate nostril breathing
Poses (Appendix D): Sun salutation, triangle pose, twisting triangle pose, revolving side angle pose, straight leg seated spinal twist, cobra pose, bow pose, bridge pose, wheel pose, shoulderstand, plough pose, relaxation pose

Insomnia

What is Insomnia?

Insomnia includes difficulty falling asleep, waking frequently throughout the night, or waking in the early morning with the inability to get back to sleep. Nearly half of all patients receiving treatment for cancer experience difficulty falling or staying asleep during cancer therapy. Sleep evaluations (polysomnograms) measure brain wave activity, eye movements, muscle tone, heart rate, breathing rate, and oxygen levels during sleep, and are sometimes used to diagnose sleep disorders.

There are many causes of insomnia in patients undergoing treatment for cancer. Certain medications such as sedatives, hypnotics, and anticonvulsants, chemotherapy, radiation, or hormonal therapy can cause sleep disturbances. Other factors such as pain, hot flashes, nausea and vomiting, irregular sleep patterns, and lifestyle (excessive napping, watching television in bed, or spending too much time in bed) can also affect sleep patterns. Women, older adults, patients with a personal or family history of insomnia, and patients with a history of depression or an anxiety disorder are at higher risk for developing insomnia.

How is Insomnia Treated by Conventional Medicine?

Treatment of insomnia includes attention to contributing factors such as pain management, hot flashes, or nausea and vomiting. Improved sleep may be promoted by adopting sleep hygiene behaviors such as changing the sleeping environment to reduce interruptions, establishing and maintaining a bedtime and a wake time, avoiding stimulants such as caffeine containing beverages, and exercising on a consistent basis (as little as three 20-minute sessions per week) at least six hours before bedtime. Cognitive-behavioral, relaxation training, and stimulus control techniques may also be beneficial. The use of sleep medications such as benzodiazepines, hypnotics, antihistamines, and tricyclic antidepressants may be prescribed. Caution is advised with these agents as they may lead to excessive next-day sleepiness, dependence, and rebound insomnia once discontinued.

Integrative Approaches to Insomnia

General strategies such as avoiding overly stimulating visual and audio images such as, television, radio, computer use, or gaming, avoiding bright lights, using dimmed lights in the evening, and avoiding heavy lifting and high-impact exercise in the evening. Many integrative therapies appeal to sensory emotions and elicit feelings of relaxation and comfort. For mild cases of insomnia, begin with visualization and yogic deep breathing techniques. For patients who can exercise, low impact forms of exercise are recommended during the day. Gentle massage will often leave patients with feelings of relaxation and sleepiness during or immediately after the massage. Both acupressure and reflexology are convenient therapies that can be applied in any setting. An herbal tea before bedtime can be an evening ritual, and aromatherapy can be used on the pillow to promote sleepiness throughout the night. The nutrition recommendations may be used to manage insomnia. For severe cases of insomnia, supplementation may be beneficial.

Before adding any integrative therapy to your treatment plan, speak with your doctor about the benefits and risks. A summary of risks may be found in the Introduction along with detailed instructions for the application of and considerations for each of the indicated therapies.

Integrative Medicine in Action

Patient Story
Integrative Medicine Plan for Insomnia:
Aromatherapy, Supplements, and Visual Imagery.
Patient: Lucas, a 15-year old adolescent with Acute Lymphoblastic Leukemia experiencing insomnia.
Chief Complaint: Within a week of receiving his cancer diagnosis, Lucas could not sleep through the night. When Lucas began to receive high-dose dexamethasone as part of his chemotherapy regimen, he would lay in bed for hours struggling to fall asleep.
Treatment: Lucas followed his pediatric oncologist's suggestion of adhering to a bedtime of 10 p.m. and a wake time of 8 a.m. At some point in the day but not at bedtime, he would play interactive video sports games. At bedtime, Lucas would either dispense a few drops of lavender essential oil on his pillow case or spray a mist of bergamot essential oil throughout his room. At bedtime, he practiced deep breathing and went through a relaxing visual imagery exercise. Lucas also began taking melatonin every evening.
Outcome: Lucas began to feel in command of his ability to fall and stay asleep.

Aromatherapy

The fragrance of essential oils can calm the mind and ease you into a restful sleep. Establish a sleep regimen using essential oils before bedtime. Whether using the essential oils in a bath or through diffusion, the fragrance of the oils can relay to your mind that it is time to go to bed. Instructions for application of aromatherapy may be found in Chapter 4.

Bath/Foot bath: Geranium, Lavender, Roman chamomile, Rose
Diffusion/Direct inhalation: Bergamot, Lavender, Orange, Roman chamomile
Massage/Reflexology: Bergamot, Lavender, Roman chamomile, Rose
Mist: Bergamot, Lavender, Orange, Roman chamomile, Rose, Sweet marjoram, Ylang ylang
Special Applications
• Directly apply Lavender while massaging the back of the neck (refer to the massage section in this chapter).

Chinese Medicine/Acupressure

Insomnia refers to a variety of symptoms relating to abnormal and insufficient sleep. These include difficulty falling asleep, inability to stay asleep, waking frequently, excessive dreaming, and restlessness. There are many factors which can impact sleep in Chinese medicine theory. For example, the spirit, which resides in the heart, is susceptible to many influences, most notably heat. Since it is the nature of heat to rise, when there is excess heat in the body, it can result in too much heat in the heart and agitate the spirit. When the spirit is disrupted, it is unable to quiet at night and sleep may become difficult.

It is important for the body to receive an adequate amount of rest, particularly during treatment for cancer. Chinese medicine treatment involves calming the spirit to promote sleep and addressing any underlying and contributing condition. Using the following points throughout the day can help promote relaxation, but be sure to use them prior to going to sleep each night.

Acupressure
Most frequently used (Appendix A)
An Mian, HT 7, Yin Tang*

It can also be very effective to apply acupressure along the UB channel of the back (Appendix A).

If it is difficult to fall asleep due to anxiety, add: HT 5, PC 7, SP 6
If person wakes up frequently during the night and is restless, add: Kid 3, Liv 2, SP 6
If talking in sleep or sleepwalking during the night, add: Liv 3, PC 5

---

*Rub lightly in an upward direction.

If having excessive, vivid dreams or nightmares, add: HT 8, UB 15
If waking with sudden anxiety and palpitations, add: GB 40, PC 7
If accompanied by acid reflux, fullness in the belly & belching, add: PC 6, Ren 12, ST 36

Herbal Teas

Herbal teas, as part of an evening ritual, may help alleviate insomnia. Choose the herbal tea that is most appealing to your taste and aromatic senses. Relax with a cup of tea in the evening. Instructions for tea preparation may be found in Chapter 4.

• German chamomile (*Matricaria recutita*). Seep 1 to 2 tsp in 6 to 8 ounces of warm water for 5 to 10 minutes, strain.
• Valerian (*Valeriana officinalis*), Lemon balm (*Melissa officinalis*), and Passion flower (*Passiflora incarnate*). Mix 1 to 2 tsp of each herb in 8 ounces boiling water, seep 5 to 10 minutes, and strain.

Homeopathy

Homeopathic remedies may be taken as individual remedies (Coffea) or as mixtures of remedies (Nervoheel® N and Neurexan®). Clinical trials suggest that homeopathic mixtures may be effective in managing insomnia. Homeopathic remedies should be administered 3 times per day with the last dose 30 minutes prior to bedtime. If sleep does not improve within 2 to 3 days, consider another remedy or integrative therapy.

• Coffea. This remedy is especially good if you are experiencing an overactive mind and racing thoughts that prevent you from falling asleep.
• Nervoheel® N and Neurexan® are mixtures of homeopathic remedies that have been demonstrated to improve sleep patterns in small clinical trials. Consider either of these remedies for relief from insomnia.

Massage

Gentle massage is preferred over techniques like deep tissue massage that can stimulate circulation and make you more alert. Include massage as part of an evening ritual and add aromatherapy as this will increase the benefits. Information on the recommended massage techniques may be found in Chapter 4.

Massage by a Caregiver

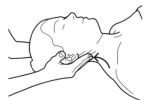

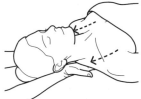

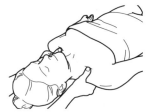

1 Have the person lie down on their back. Apply cream, lotion, or oil with aromatherapy on your hands. Begin with strokes on the back of the neck using a gliding petrissage motion and moving from the bottom of the neck up to the skull.

2 Put your hands under the person's shoulders and upper back with your palms facing up. Pull or rake your hands upward towards the head. Repeat this stroke 3 – 4 times.

3 Apply circular petrissage motions on the upper chest area above the breasts and below the collar bones on the pectoralis major muscle.

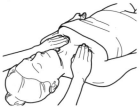

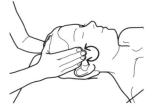

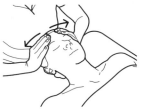

4 Press with your palms facing down on the upper chest area and move your hands in a circular motion. The goal of this technique is to enhance deep breathing.

5 Apply a small amount of cream to your fingertips. Gently press against the temples and move the fingers in small circles.

6 Put your fingers at against the forehead and pull in an outward direction towards the ears.

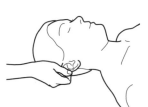

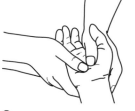

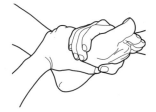

7 Gently massage the ears with slight pulling motions.

8 Begin massaging the palms and fingers.

9 Finish by massaging both feet using a grasping technique and small petrissage strokes.

10 Repeat as needed before bedtime.

Self Massage

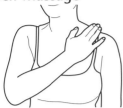 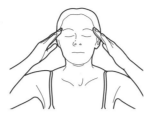

1 Put some lotion or cream blended with aromatherapy oil on your hands. Take the right palm of your hand and massage the left side of your chest above the breast but below the collar bone. Repeat with your left palm on the right side of your chest.

2 Massage your temples with small circular petrissage motions. Avoid the eye area to prevent cream or oil from entering the eye.

3 Repeat these steps several times a day as needed, particularly before bedtime.

Nutrition

Nutrition alone is not likely to entirely manage insomnia but will help promote restful sleep when combined with other integrative therapies, particularly aromatherapy or any of the touch therapies. Dietary patterns such as avoiding eating late at night (your last meal should be 2 to 3 hours prior to bedtime) and choosing small portions (avoid overeating in the late afternoon and evening) may also be beneficial.

Foods to Avoid

• Caffeine-rich beverages and food. Try decaffeinated varieties of both coffee and tea, and avoid chocolate during periods of severe insomnia. Eliminate energy-boosting drinks from your dietary plan.

• Alcohol. Limit or eliminate alcohol consumption.

• Avoid meals high in saturated fat ("bad fat") in the evening. Emphasize lean portions of protein such as fish, poultry, and turkey.

Foods to Emphasize

• L-tryptophan is a natural sedative. High levels of l-tryptophan are found in turkey. Other foods rich in l-tryptophan include chicken, milk, cheese, cow's milk yogurt, beans, and cashews.

Quick Dietary Tips

• Avoid late-night overeating and exercising
• Emphasize foods high in l-tryptophan
• Avoid heavy alcohol consumption

- Complex carbohydrates. Brown rice, quinoa, bran, and whole-grain oats should be included in your diet. Avoid refined carbohydrates.
- Drink warm milk 30 to 45 minutes before bedtime.

Reflexology

Reflexology can enhance relaxation by calming the nervous system and releasing endorphins. It can be applied any time during the day; however, around bedtime is optimal. When the feet are relaxed the mind and body can relax. Information on reflexology technique may be found in Chapter 4.

Foot Points
R: Adrenal reflexes
T: Diaphragm, lung, solar plexus, spinal reflexes; neck/shoulder line

Hand Points
R: Adrenal reflexes
T: Lung, solar plexus, spinal reflexes; all the fingers

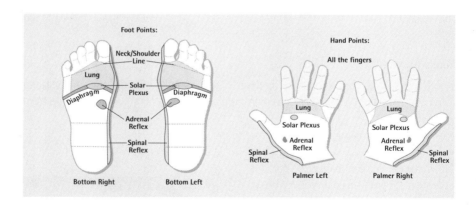

Supplements

Many of the supplements listed below have been evaluated in clinical trials; however, some such as melatonin and valerian interact with certain chemotherapy agents and must be avoided if you are receiving treatment with these drugs. Herbal teas may be a better option during cancer therapy. Speak with your doctor about whether or not supplements are safe during your cancer therapy.

- **Melatonin.** 3 to 5 mg per day, administered in the evening, 45 minutes before bedtime.
- Valerian (*Valeriana spp*). Often combined with other herbal supplements to provide a sedative effect. Start with valerian at a dose of 400 to 900 mg per day, 2 hours prior to bedtime. If no relief is obtained after 2 to 4 weeks of administration, add other sedative herbal remedies:

You may choose 1 to 3 depending on your condition.

- Lemon balm (*Melissa officinalis*). 395 mg per day.
- Passion flower (*Passiflora incarnata*). 300 to 400 mg per day.
- Hops (*Humulus lupulus*). 1 to 2 grams per day.

Visual Imagery

This visual imagery will work best if you are lying down in your bed for the night. If you need to set your alarm for the morning, do it at this point. Turn off any noise. Lie on your back in a comfortable position.

Start with the feet. Become aware of your feet. Tighten up your feet as hard as you can. Then let go. Feel the toes, the arches and the heels let go and start to relax. Now tighten up your legs. Now let go. Feel the muscles in your calves, around your knees, and in your thighs get heavy. Imagine they are sinking into the bed. Feel them relax with every breath.

Now tighten up your lower belly. Now let go. Feel your belly relaxing with every breath. Feel your breath traveling down into the belly as you inhale. Exhale any tension you might be feeling in this area. Now tighten up your hands and arms as tight as you can. Now let them go. Let them drop with heaviness onto the bed. Feel the tension in the hands, the wrists, the forearms, elbows, upper arms, and shoulders let go with relaxation.

Now bring your inhalation into the chest. Feel your ribs expand as you inhale. Feel all the tension in the chest area let go with your exhalation. Repeat three times. Now tighten up your face as tight as you can. Now let go. Feel the jaw relax. Feel the cheeks relax. Feel the forehead relax. Feel your eyes relax.

Now, just focus on your breath. As you inhale, imagine your whole body filling up like a balloon. Gently let the air out of this "balloon" through your mouth. Repeat this five times. Tell yourself that with every exhale you fall deeper and deeper into relaxation. Tell yourself by the tenth breath you will be fully and soundly asleep. Let yourself drift off. Tell yourself that you will sleep through the night and wake up in the morning fully refreshed and energized.

Yoga

Yoga aims to prepare your body for sleep. Yoga relaxes the mind, soothes the muscles, and quiets the breath. The suggested yoga routine should be practiced within one hour before going to sleep.

Breathing (Appendix D): Ujjayi breath, alternate nostril breathing
Poses (Appendix D): Chair pose, tree pose, standing forward bend, relaxation pose

Loss of Appetite

What is Loss of Appetite?

Loss of appetite is eating less than usual, not being hungry, or feeling full after eating only a small amount of food. A poor appetite during cancer treatment can result in malnutrition, loss of muscle mass, weight loss, and cachexia.

Loss of appetite can be caused by cancer or by cancer therapy. Chemotherapy; radiation therapy to the head and neck, esophagus, stomach or intestines; feeling of fullness from fluid collection in the belly; and use of sedative medications are examples of therapies that might cause loss of appetite. Some side effects of cancer treatments such as nausea and vomiting and change in taste and smell can also contribute to loss of appetite.

Persistent loss of appetite can lead to cachexia, a severe form of malnutrition. Cachexia is a syndrome and is associated with changes in basal metabolism and biological processes that further depress appetite and make eating difficult.

How is Loss of Appetite Treated by Conventional Medicine?

Appetite should improve when the underlying side effects that are causing the loss of appetite are effectively managed. Medications that stimulate the appetite (Marinol®, megestrol acetate or Megace®, dexamethasone), nutritional supplements (Ensure®), and advanced forms of nutrition intervention (nasogastric tubes, gastrostomy tubes, total parenteral nutrition) are some of the standard treatments available for loss of appetite. However, these interventions cannot entirely manage loss of appetite. Consultation with a nutritionist or registered dietician prior to and throughout the cancer treatment may help prevent persistent loss of appetite and weight loss.

Integrative Approaches to Loss of Appetite

Integrative therapies works best for early symptoms of loss of appetite. If you are experiencing substantial weight loss due to loss of appetite, your doctor will likely prescribe advanced forms of nutrition intervention. If you are just beginning to experience loss of appetite, your goal should be to maintain your current weight and appetite. Begin with conventional and integrative dietary changes that are easiest for you to adopt. You may also want to consider supplements to avoid further declines in weight. If you are experiencing loss of appetite that has persisted for weeks to months, choose a supplement along with other therapies. For example, aromatherapy and herbal teas can stimulate your senses and enhance salivation, thereby making food choices more enticing.

Work with your doctor to choose the best supplement. Often, supplements can be combined with an appetite stimulant. If your loss of appetite is associated with another side effect, refer to the associated chapter for additional integrative interventions.

Before adding any integrative therapy to your treatment plan, speak with your doctor about the benefits and risks. A summary of risks may be found in the Introduction along with detailed instructions for the application of and considerations for each of the indicated therapies.

Integrative Medicine in Action

Patient Story
Integrative Medicine Plan for Loss of Appetite:
Herbal Teas and Nutrition.
Patient: Alexandria, a 61-year old woman with lung cancer experiencing loss of appetite.
Chief Complaint: After three months of chemotherapy and radiation, Alexandria had no appetite at all. Alexandria described food as tasting funny and she was afraid to eat. The appetite stimulants prescribed by her doctor were not helping to increase her appetite.
Treatment: Alexandria and her husband met with a registered dietician to develop a plan to help her maintain her weight. Weekly grocery lists and meal plans were prepared one week in advance and were modified as her tastes changed. The grocery list included a variety of nuts and nut butters, avocados, salmon, and pineapple. She also chose eggs and cereal products that were fortified with Omega 3 fatty acids. Every day her husband would also make her a calorie-rich smoothie. He also made a bitter orange tea, which he gave her a half-hour before her meals.
Outcome: Through counseling, Alexandria and her husband were able to come up with meal plans consisting of nutrient dense foods she could enjoy. She only gained a few pounds after initiating the diet changes, but she was able to prevent any further weight loss throughout her remaining cancer treatment.

Aromatherapy

Comfort smells can provoke feelings of hunger much like the smell of a bakery or the smell of your favorite food being prepared. Choose an appealing aroma and use throughout the day with any application. Instructions for application of aromatherapy may be found in Chapter 4.

Diffusion/Direct Inhalation: Bergamot, Ginger, Orange
Mist: Bergamot, Orange
If Loss of Appetite is due to Taste Changes:
Diffusion/Direct Inhalation: Basil, Helichrysum, Peppermint
Mist: Peppermint

Special Applications
• Directly apply Ginger or Orange on acupressure point ST 36 (Appendix A).

Chinese Medicine/Acupressure

In TCM, a decrease in appetite is caused by a disharmony of the spleen and stomach. The stomach processes the food and fluids we eat while the spleen transforms food and fluids into nutrients and makes them available throughout the body. When the spleen and stomach are functioning properly and the digestive qi is balanced, the body can easily break down and absorb the food we eat. Furthermore, hunger is felt at regular intervals and typical size meals can be enjoyed without bloating, discomfort, nausea, or vomiting. If the stomach and/or spleen are unable to properly process food, then a decrease in appetite and/or feelings of fullness will be easily felt after eating only a small amount of food.

Acupressure
Most frequently used (Appendix A)
Ren 11, Ren 12, SP 3, SP 4, ST 36
Taste Changes
Changes in taste are associated with many different TCM patterns and may also contribute to loss of appetite. The kind of taste change will determine the underlying disharmony and treatment approach. Use the acupoints that most reflect your changes in taste. For example, if you find foods taste very sweet or not sweet enough, use the acupoints associated with "sweet" tastes.

• **Bitter:** GB 34, Liv 2, Liv 3
• **Sweet:** Ren 12, SP 3, ST 36
• **Salty:** Kid 3, Kid 6
• **Sour:** Liv 3, SP 6
• **Bland (refers to a decrease in the overall sense of taste in the mouth):** Ren 12, SP 9, ST 36

Herbal Teas

Digestive bitters and warming teas may help stimulate the appetite. Bitter teas should be taken at least 20 minutes before a meal or snack. Choose the flavor that is most appealing to you. Instructions for tea preparation may be found in Chapter 4.

- Bitter orange (*Citrus aurantium*). 1 to 2 teaspoons in 6 to 8 ounces of hot water, seep for 10 minutes, strain.
- Dandelion (*Taraxacum officinale*). 1 to 2 teaspoons of herb in 6 to 8 ounces of boiling water, seep for 15 minutes, strain. Add 1 to 2 teaspoons of Gentian (*Gentiana lutea)* or tangerine peel for an additive effect. Honey or agave nectar will sweeten the flavor.
- Ginger (*Zingiber officinale*). Grate fresh ginger, add 1/2 to1 tsp of grated ginger to warm water, seep for 5 to 10 minutes (for a stronger flavor, seep longer), strain. Add one teaspoon of honey to sweeten the flavor. Drink throughout the day.
- Tangerine peel. Seep 2 to 4 thin slices of tangerine peel in 6 to 8 ounces of hot water for 5 to 10 minutes (depending on strength desired). If tangerine is not appealing, you may also try dried orange peel.

Nutrition

Managing loss of appetite before you begin to lose weight will help you tolerate the side effects of chemotherapy. Your doctor can advise you as to which points in your therapy may cause you to experience decreased appetite. A nutritionist or registered dietician can then help you develop and prioritize strategies to manage decreased appetite in order to avoid weight loss. Strive to stay within 5% of your weight at diagnosis. If you have already experienced weight loss or gain, your goal should be weight management. Focus on remediating weight loss or weight gain when your cancer treatment is complete.

Simple strategies to prevent weight loss:

- Eat throughout the day.
- Eat small, but frequent meals and snacks.
- Choose nutrient-dense foods (foods with a lot of nutrients and calories per bite); however, do not confuse this with eating unhealthy nutrient dense foods such as fried foods.
- Avoid empty calories such as soda, juice, and refined bread and snack products.
- Maintain your social network and eat out with friends.

A daily menu plan can remove the anxiety or stress of meal planning. Engage close friends and family to shop for groceries, prepare meals, and manage your dietary schedule. Prepare and freeze food to lessen the burden of food preparation and weekly meal planning.

Other conditions associated with cancer treatment can affect your appetite such as nausea and vomiting (refer to this chapter for specific recommendations). Speak with your doctor if your weight is making you frustrated and overwhelmed. In certain

circumstances advanced nutrition interventions may be necessary to maintain
your weight and nutrition status. Your
doctor or nutritionist may recommend
a feeding tube or some other form of
advanced nutrition support. Most often,
advanced nutrition interventions are
temporary and enable patients to maintain weight during therapy and relieve the
anxiety, stress, and frustration associated
with weight loss.

Quick Dietary Tips

• Prepare for loss of appetite. Speak with your doctor to identify highest risk periods
• Eat small amounts frequently
• Choose nutrient dense foods as fuel for your body

Food Remedies

• Avoid "plain" foods. Increase your calories by adding spreads, sauces, or dips to any food. For example, celery sticks with almond or cashew butter are an alternative to plain celery sticks.
• Eat a variety of foods. It is easier to eat more food when variety is available. When eating out, choose several appetizers for your meal rather than a single entrée. Choose variety over monotony at every meal.
• Eat "good" fats (Omega 3 and 6). Choose eggs, cereal, and pasta products enriched with Omega 3. Use canned salmon, extra virgin olive oil, and flax seed oil for dressings. Choose nuts (macadamia, walnuts, cashews, pistachios, almonds) and avocados throughout the day.
• Make a protein-packed smoothie each day. In a blender, mix the following:

   o 30 to 50 grams of whey protein powder (about 1 to 2 scoops depending on the product)
   o 1 cup of nut butter (almond, macadamia, cashew; avoid peanut)
   o 1 cup of full fat yogurt (Greek yogurt)
   o 1 cup of fresh berries
   o 1 tbsp agave nectar
   o 1 to 2 tbsp flaxseed oil, essential fatty acid oil, or medium chain triglyceride oil
   o 1/2 cup shredded coconut
   o 1 to 1 1/2 banana (add more banana for a thicker consistency)
   o 1/2 cup to 1 cup of milk (dairy, soy, or rice). You can also use meal replacements such as Ensure® instead of milk for added calories.

• Add pineapple and grapefruit to your diet. Both these remedies are common in TCM. Grapefruit can interfere with some medications so speak with your doctor before adding to your diet.

- A small glass of white or red wine (3 ounces) can increase the appetite. Speak with your doctor before drinking alcohol during your therapy.
- Many herbs are traditionally used to engage the appetite. Enjoy foods prepared with basil, fennel, coriander, ginger, fenugreek, turmeric, anise, cinnamon, tarragon, onion, rosemary, or sage.

Reflexology

The recommended points are linked to organs that promote hunger and aid with digestion. Stimulate the points throughout the day or as needed. Information on reflexology technique may be found in Chapter 4.

Foot Points
F: Mouth, throat reflexes
H: Hypothalamus, pituitary, reflexes
T: Esophagus, stomach reflexes

Hand Points
F: Mouth reflexes
H: Hypothalamus, pituitary reflexes
T: Esophagus, stomach, throat reflexes

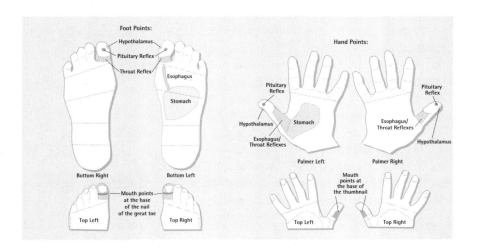

Supplements

Essential fatty acids or whey protein may increase your appetite, similar to appetite stimulants. Medium chain triglyceride oil can enhance the absorption of calories. Most of these supplements can be used in combination with conventional strategies to help manage loss of appetite. Begin with essential fatty acids, and consider medium chain triglyceride oil for additional calories.

• **Essential fatty acids (fish oils).** 4 to 6 grams per day of a mixture of eicosapentanoic acid (EPA) and docosahexaenoic acid (DHA). Lower doses of fatty acids are not effective for appetite stimulation. Choose supplements that provide approximately 60% EPA/40% DHA. **High doses of fish oils should not be used if you have problems with blood clotting.** Consult with your doctor before using essential fatty acids.
• Medium chain triglyceride (MCT) oil. 1 to 3 tablespoons per day. MCT can be taken with food, added to a smoothie, or taken alone. The type of fats found in coconut, coconut oil, palm kernel oil, and MCT oil are easily digested when compared to other fats and are frequently used for patients with chronic diarrhea and other malabsorption disorders. MCT oil is available with a prescription or over the counter. Consult with your doctor before using MCT oil if you have a liver disorder or diabetes.
• Whey protein. 30 to 50 grams per day depending on the product. Whey is a protein concentrate extracted from the protein solids found in milk. Whey protein may be added to a wide variety of foods and beverages without altering the taste. If you have milk allergies, do an allergy test before using whey.

Visual Imagery

Sit up in a chair with your spine straight. Close your eyes and take several deep breaths. Imagine your body relaxing with every breath. Each breath you take should be deeper and deeper. Eventually you want your belly to expand as you inhale. When you feel as though your mind and body are relaxed through the breaths (this could take from 10 to 20 minutes), bring your focus to the area right below your belly button. Imagine this area is a fireplace. Visualize a calming and gentle fire crackling in the imaginary fireplace inside your belly just below your belly button. This fire is warming to the belly. It's comfortable. Feel this fire gently and comfortably warming up your lower belly. Feel this warm feeling in the front of your body and your lower back. This gentle fire is warming both the front and back of you.

Imagine that this fire is bringing movement to your belly. You can imagine a gurgling sensation or growling or wave-like movements behind your belly button. As the fire increases, the gurgling increases. You feel yourself getting hungry. Stay with this image until you feel any slight sensation of hunger.

Now picture what you are hungry for. If you can't think of anything, pick your favorite food. See it in front of you. Imagine what it might smell like. The imaginary smell makes you hungrier. You might even hear more gurgling in your stomach. Feel your mouth salivating for this food. Feel the cravings increase as your visualization becomes clearer and clearer. See yourself eating the food and enjoying every bite. Imagine that this food is the tastiest it's ever been. Imagine that it's dissolving in your mouth and exploding on your palate.

At your own pace, open your eyes and go get the food that you just imagined or any food you might have that will satisfy you.

Yoga

Use yoga to support digestion, improve metabolism, and enhance relaxation. The combination of yoga poses targeting these areas is ideal during those time periods when you do not feel hungry or are eating less than usual.

Breathing (Appendix D): Ujjayi breath, kapalabhati
Poses (Appendix D): Prayer twist, seated forward bend, relaxation pose

Loss of Libido

What is Loss of Libido?

The loss of libido, one of the most common sexual problems affecting both men and women with cancer, is described as the loss of desire, interest, or motivation for sexual activity. Loss of libido may not resolve during cancer treatment and may linger throughout the first few years following the completion of cancer treatment.

Many types of cancer and cancer treatment can cause physical, physiological, and psychological problems which impact the ability to function sexually and lessen sexual desire. Some cancer treatments, such as hormone therapy, decrease sexual desire by disturbing a normal hormone balance. Some surgeries, such as mastectomies for breast cancer and radical prostatectomies for prostate cancer, may directly affect sexual function, contributing to a lack of sexual desire. Chemotherapy associated side effects such as hair loss, weight gain or loss, nausea and vomiting, mouth sores, constipation, and diarrhea can also alter sexual self image and self esteem. Fear and anxiety may cause avoidance of intimacy, touch, and sexual activity. Depression, resulting from changes in physical appearance from cancer treatment, may lead to feelings of unattractiveness.

How is Loss of Libido Treated by Conventional Medicine?

Loss of libido may improve when underlying conditions are addressed. It is important for patients and their partners to discuss the loss of sexual desire with a health care professional to learn how to effectively deal with these problems. Both medical and psychological approaches are recommended. Treatment approaches include sexual counseling, hormone replacements, and lifestyle changes which manage stress and anxiety and rebuild self esteem.

Integrative Approaches to Loss of Libido

The integrative approach is to clear the mind of chatter or distractions and enhance the innate senses (touch, smell and sound). By accomplishing this, you will feel less inhibited and more open to experience feelings of sensuality, sexuality, or sexual arousal. In this chapter, we focus on touch therapies combined with aromatherapy, couples yoga breath and movement, and visual imagery. Use these therapies in any environment that appeals to you.

Before adding any integrative therapy to your treatment plan, speak with your doctor about the benefits and risks. A summary of risks may be found in the Introduction along with detailed instructions for the application of and considerations for each of the indicated therapies.

Integrative Medicine in Action

Patient Story
Integrative Medicine Plan for Loss of Libido:
Massage, Visual Imagery, and Yoga.
Patient: Doug, a 46-year old man with prostate cancer experiencing loss of libido.
Chief Complaint: One year after his radical prostatectomy, Doug's erectile dysfunction that came about as a result of his surgery began to resolve. Although now sexually able, his motivation for sex was limited by his poor self image. Doug became depressed and felt inadequate.
Treatment: Doug's wife encouraged him to speak to his oncologist about his lack of sexual motivation. At his next doctor's visit, Doug's oncologist referred him for sexual counseling. During one of his sexual counseling sessions, the therapist encouraged him to quiet his mind and use visual imagery. Doug followed a recorded script for a few weeks. His wife's massage therapist suggested couples massage, and taught her some basic techniques to do at home. Setting the mood for romantic evenings, Doug and his wife would turn off their phones and dim the lights. Doug and his wife used this peaceful time together to also practice partner-assisted yoga.
Outcome: Through sexual counseling and creation of an intimate environment with his wife, Doug was able to rebuild his feelings of adequacy. Doug felt his desire for sex return through consistent practice of visual imagery, partner-assisted yoga, and massage.

Aromatherapy

Fragrance can have a powerful effect on sexual desire. Diffusing or massaging a pleasant essential oil on your body can instill a sense of wanting to be touched and enhance sexual stimulation. Instructions for application of aromatherapy may be found in Chapter 4.

Direct Application/Direct Inhalation/Massage: Black pepper, Cinnamon, Ginger, Rose, Ylang ylang. Massage should be directed to lower belly, neck, back, and ankles.
Special Applications
• Directly apply any of the above essential oils on acupressure points (refer to the acupressure section in this chapter).
• To set the mood and environment for creating sexual intimacy, diffuse Cinnamon or Orange essential oil.

Chinese Medicine/Acupressure

According to Chinese medicine, the Kidney yang is the source of sexual desire. The Kidney yang is the warming, activating force which stimulates both sexual desire and function. It can be injured by long term illness or exposure to treatments such as chemotherapy and radiation.

Acupressure can be used to stimulate the Kidney yang and increase libido particularly when used right before or during a sexual encounter. By stimulating the lower Ren and the Liver channels, acupressure can boost the kidney yang and promote qi and blood flow through the sexual organs. These points can be stimulated alone or with a partner.

Acupressure
Most frequently used (Appendix A)
Kid 7, Liv 5, Ren 1
Secondary points (Appendix A)
HT 7, Liv 8, Liv 10, Ren 2, ST 30

Massage

Massage therapy can enhance feelings of deep relaxation thereby calming the mind and allowing feeling of sexuality to arise. By massaging the whole body, one can elicit stimulation of the nerve endings at the level of the skin and muscles. Use all strokes starting with long effleurage strokes on the back, buttocks and legs. Adding aromatherapy to the massage can boost feelings of sexuality. Information on the recommended massage techniques may be found in Chapter 4.

Massage by a Caregiver

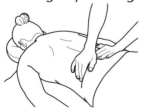 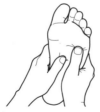 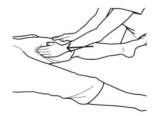

1 Apply small massage to the back, buttocks and legs by using smaller circular and grasping petrissage technique. Linger over the areas that feel best on the person.

2 Have the person lie down on their back. Apply petrissage strokes to the feet. Use two hands for one foot. Massage the bottom and then the top of the feet. Apply lighter pressure to boney areas such as the ankle bones and the top of the feet.

3 Use long strokes moving upward on the inner thighs. The muscles in this area attach to the lower pelvis bone. By massaging the adductor and internal rotator muscles, this can elicit relaxation and/or stimulation to the pelvic area.

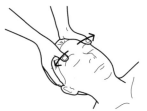 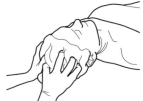

4 Lightly massage the face. Circle the eyes and massage the jaw area with light strokes. Use a light thumb stroke over the frontalis muscle on the forehead.

5 Finish massaging the whole head as if you are shampooing your scalp.

Self Massage

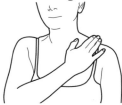 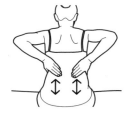 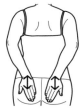

1 Use the palms of your hands and press against the upper corners of the chest by the front of the shoulders using small circular petrissage strokes. This opens up the constriction over the lungs and allows you to take deeper breaths.

2 Put your hands over your lower back area over the kidneys. Brush up and down with petrissage strokes.

3 Repeat the same brushing technique over your sacram (triangle shaped bone on the bottom of the spine) and buttocks.

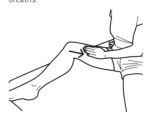 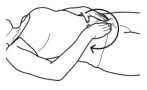

4 Starting from your knees on the inner thighs, use long effleurage strokes from the knees to the pelvis. Repeat 3 – 4 times.

5 Finish by using circular petrissage motions over the upper and lower belly. First go clockwise over the whole belly area. Make the circles big enough so you cover the muscles above the pubic bone. Repeat this in a counterclockwise motion.

Nutrition

Throughout history, several foods have been promoted to improve sexual desire. Foods retaining this quality are frequently referred to as aphrodisiacs. Most modern day aphrodisiac foods date back to ancient Greek and Egyptian times and are a component of both Ayurvedic and TCM. These medical systems have a long history of combining herbs, tonics, and foods to promote sexual desire.

Being creative in the presentation and serving of the foods may make them more appealing. For example, serve strawberries, pineapple, raspberries, and apples with chocolate fondue rather than a chocolate bar. Drizzle honey and chocolate on sliced apples, pineapples, or strawberries instead of serving them plain. Oysters, a hallmark of aphrodisiac foods, can be enjoyed grilled, on a half shell, broiled, smoked, or added to stews or chowders; however, avoid raw oysters if you are experiencing neutropenia. Enjoy a glass of wine as an aperitif with your partner. Be creative and try variation!

Foods that Promote Sexual Desire
Apples, Almonds, Caviar, Chocolate, Chili Peppers, Honey, Eggs, Milk, Pineapples, Oysters, Strawberries, Raspberries with Whipped Cream, Grapes, Vanilla, Truffles, Pumpkin Seeds, Mint, Ginger Root, Rosemary, Figs, Peaches, Mango, Nuts, and Saffron.

Reflexology

In reflexology, the feet are considered an erogenous zone. Stimulating these points can remove inhibitions and create synergistic energy. Reflexology can also be applied simultaneously between partners. Reflexology, like massage, acupressure, and partner-assisted yoga are all touch therapies that can create a physical connection with your partner. Information on reflexology technique may be found in Chapter 4.

Foot Points
F: Fallopian tube/vas deferens reflexes
R: Adrenals, ovary/teste, uterus/prostate reflexes
T: Diaphragm line, lung, solar plexus, spinal reflexes

Hand Points
F: All the fingers
H: Pituitary reflexes
R: Ovary/teste, uterus/prostate reflexes
T: Solar plexus, spinal reflexes

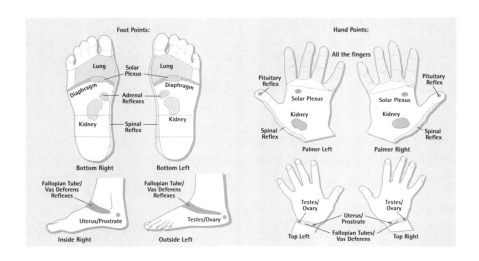

Visual Imagery

Sit up with your spine straight. Focus on your breath. As you inhale, imagine the breath relaxing all your muscles. As you exhale, image all the tension, pain or any uncomfortable feelings leave with the breath. Inhale, the muscles relax, exhale and all tension leaves with the breath. Repeat five times.

Focus on your spine. Feel the end of the spine or coccyx area, where it meets the chair. Imagine a color of red at the base of your spine. Feel that color stimulating the local area at the base. When the area begins to feel tingling or warm move up the spine to the lower back. Now imagine a color of orange filling up your lower back area. If you can, in the back of your mind, know that the red color is still at the base as you're creating the orange area in the lower back. Feel this area start to tingle. Even if you don't feel it, imagine what it would feel like as if the color is stimulating the area.

Once that is achieved, move up the spine to thsse middle of the back. Imagine a color of yellow filling up the middle back. Again, stay with this imagery until you feel the warmth or tingling feeling in the middle area of your back. Now move up to the upper back area in between the shoulder blades. Imagine a green light. Stay with this imagery until you feel warmth or tingling in the area. Move up the spine to the back of the neck. See a blue light opening up the throat. In the back of your mind, you are still seeing the red light at the base, the orange light at the lower back, the yellow light in the mid back and the green light in the upper back. All of these colors up to the blue light in the throat provide stimulation to the spine.

Feel the tingling sensation going up and down the spine. With this tingling feeling, allow yourself to feel aroused.

Repeat as needed.

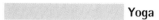 **Yoga**

Complement your own yoga routine by practicing partner-assisted yoga. This can be a great way to connect with your spouse or partner in an intimate way. Set the mood for partner-assisted yoga by wearing comfortable clothing in an appealing environment.

Breathing (Appendix D): Ujjayi breath, alternate nostril breathing, kapalabhati
Poses (Appendix D): Cobbler's pose (opens genitals and heightens sensitivity in the area), legs up relaxation pose, relaxation pose

To come into the suggested poses with your partner, refer to the following instructions:

1. Come to sit in Cobbler's pose. Facing your partner, sit 2 to 3 feet away from each other. Reach forward and grab your partner's hands. Then pull your partner forward to come into the full pose. Take 5 deep breaths. When your partner is ready, have your partner pull you forward to come into the full pose. Take 5 deep breaths. Repeat.
2. Come into the Legs up relaxation pose by sitting with your buttocks against your partner's buttocks. Use each other as a wall. Reach forward and grab your partner's hands. Breathe deeply together for 5 to 10 minutes.
3. Holding hands with your partner, lie back into Relaxation pose. Lying together, breathe deeply for 10 minutes.

Lymphedema

What is Lymphedema?

Lymphedema is swelling in the soft tissues of the body due to build-up of fluid from damage or blockage of the lymph system. This condition is a common problem resulting from cancer or cancer treatment and may develop following surgical removal or radiation to lymph nodes in the underarm, pelvis, groin, or neck. It can happen immediately after surgery (acute) or months to years after cancer treatment has been completed (chronic) and is usually categorized in stages (I to III) or by degree of severity (mild to severe).

Risk factors for developing lymphedema include:

• High number of lymph nodes removed. There is less risk with the removal of only the sentinel lymph node (the first node that receives lymphatic drainage from a tumor).
• Being overweight or obese.
• Slow wound healing after lymph node surgery.
• Location: A tumor that affects or blocks the left lymph duct or lymph nodes or vessels in the neck, chest, underarm, pelvis, or belly.
• Cancer Type: Breast cancer (especially if treated with breast and axillary node removal), uterine cancer, prostate cancer, lymphoma, melanoma, vulvar cancer, and ovarian cancer.

How is Lymphedema Treated by Conventional Medicine?

Prevention of lymphedema begins with education in identification of early signs of edema and with being evaluated by a certified lymphatic therapist to determine if it is possible to exercise the affected area. To help reduce symptoms of lymphedema, the following steps are recommended:

• Avoid heavy lifting.
• Elevate the affected part of the body above the level of the heart to keep lymph from pooling in the affected limb.
• Keep nails and skin clean to reduce the risk of infection.
• Stay away from hot tubs and saunas and use sunscreen to avoid getting a sunburn in the affected area.
• Avoid situations that can squeeze the involved area such as tight clothes, tight jewelry, or blood pressure cuffs.
• Avoid weight gain.

• Exercise regularly under the guidance of a certified fitness professional or physical therapist, gradually incorporating non-fatiguing aerobic exercise and progressive weight lifting. If you do not have any signs of lymphedema, a pressure garment (also known as lymphedema sleeves or stockings) may not be needed during exercise.

Treatment of lymphedema focuses on controlling limb swelling, reducing complications associated with lymphedema, and incorporating measures that help improve your ability to perform daily activities and that support range of motion and function of the affected area. For treatment of moderate and severe cases of lymphedema, aerobic exercise; progressive weight lifting; pressure garments; bandages; physical therapy; use of a compression device, which creates a pumping action to help move fluid; weight loss; and laser therapy may be recommended. Surgery is rarely recommended. If you are experiencing lymphedema, wearing a well-fitted pressure garment during exercise that uses the affected area or limb is advised.

Integrative Approaches to Lymphedema

Integrative therapies focus on maintaining the movement of fluids through the lymphatic system. Our approach centers on touch therapies and yoga. Lymphatic drainage is the only massage technique recommended for the prevention and management of lymphedema. A simplified version of lymphatic drainage can be provided by a caregiver; however, it is recommended to also consult a licensed massage therapist specializing in Manual Lymphatic Drainage technique for ongoing therapy. Reflexology can also help move the lymph without actually touching the affected area.

Exercise is an important component in the prevention of lymphedema, specifically a progressive resistance routine and/or a mild aerobic exercise program. Heavy lifting and strenuous exercise should be avoided. Yoga can provide both aerobic and resistance exercise which promotes circulation and the flow of lymph. Supplements can either be administered topically (alone or combined with either lymphatic drainage or reflexology) or ingested. Oral supplements are best indicated as a prevention strategy after completion of cancer treatment so as to decrease the risk of a possible interaction with your conventional therapy.

Before adding any integrative therapy to your treatment plan, speak with your doctor about the benefits and risks. A summary of risks may be found in the Introduction along with detailed instructions for the application of and considerations for each of the indicated therapies.

Integrative Medicine in Action

Patient Story
Integrative Medicine Plan for Lymphedema:
Massage and Yoga.
Patient: Ana, a 34-year old woman with breast cancer experiencing lymphedema.
Chief Complaint: Ana felt that the preventive measures she was taking to avoid lymphedema following her partial mastectomy were not helping. Ana was worried that her lymphedema might become severe if she did not make additional changes during her upcoming radiation treatments. She was also worried about her recent weight gain.
Treatment: After discussing options with her oncologist, Ana found a licensed massage therapist experienced in working with cancer patients and with Manual Lymphatic Drainage technique. Ana received two massages a week for one month, one from a licensed massage therapist, and one from a caregiver. Both used the lymphatic drainage technique. Ana began practicing a 30 minute gentle yoga routine consisting of kapalabhati breathing, three rounds of sun salutations, and legs up relaxation pose during the afternoon.
Outcome: Ana was pleased that her lymphedema did not progress. Ana continued to see the massage therapist and to practice yoga on a consistent basis.

Aromatherapy

Essential oils can help improve circulation and may relieve fluid retention when incorporated into lymphatic drainage massage. The oils listed below can be used individually or combined. Instructions for application of aromatherapy may be found in Chapter 4.

Massage (lymphatic drainage): Cypress, Lemon, Rosemary. Refer to the massage section in this chapter for the recommended technique.

Homeopathy

Homeopathy may provide relief when you are experiencing lymphedema. Supplementation should continue for 6 to 8 weeks. If relief is not obtained, discontinue supplementation and consider another integrative therapy.

- Apis. 200c, once daily.

Massage

If you are currently experiencing lymphedema, massage on the affected area should be avoided.

Very light massage may be administered to unaffected parts of the body. The technique described below is lymphatic drainage and the only type of massage we suggest for patients at risk of developing or experiencing lymphedema.

Perform the sequences below the day prior to chemotherapy. Do not perform massage the day of and the two days following the chemotherapy cycle. On the third day repeat the sequence and continue until the day before your next cycle of chemotherapy. If you have completed your cancer treatment, repeat this sequence one to two times a week. Information on the recommended massage techniques can be found in Chapter 4.

Caution: Do not directly touch any area affected with lymphedema. If you are experiencing lymphedema in a certain area, skip that part of the sequence and continue with the next steps.

Massage by a Caregiver

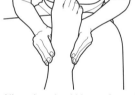 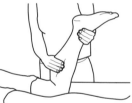 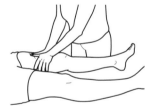

All strokes should be performed using an upward movement towards the heart.

1 The recipient of massage can either be on their back, on their belly, or on their side. They should be in the most comfortable position.

2 Begin at the ankle area by using a **light** grasping or squeezing technique.

3 With this technique, let go and grasp above the ankle.

4 Keep repeating this grasping/squeezing technique until the knee area.

5 When you get to the area above the knee use both hands on either side of the thigh and continue this grasping/squeezing technique until you reach the upper thigh.

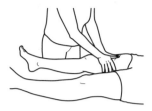

6 Repeat entire sequence on the other side, beginning at the ankle. Grasp and release all the way up to the other upper thigh.

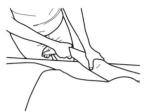

7 Start with the wrist and use the grasp/squeeze technique until the elbow.

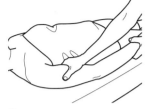

8 Use both hands now on either side of the upper arm as you grasp and squeeze up to the shoulder.

Self Massage

Self massage is not recommended for lymphedema.

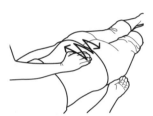

9 Have the person lie on their belly. Apply small, circular petrissage motions and massage over the entire lower back beginning at the bottom of the ribs and moving down on both sides towards the hip bones and sacrum (triangle shaped bone on the bottom of the spine). Finish with "brushing" technique over sacrum.

Supplements

Creams applied to the skin or supplements taken by mouth may assist in the prevention or management of lymphedema. Some of the supplements listed are being investigated in clinical trials. Consider topical supplements during therapy and consider oral supplements after completing your cancer treatment.

Creams applied to the skin
• Horse Chestnut (*Aesculus hippocastanum*). Gentle application to affected area, 1 to 2 times per day. Creams can be combined with either lymphatic drainage or reflexology.

Oral

• Horse Chestnut (*Aesculus hippocastanum*). Apsules are standardized to aescin, the active ingredient in horse chestnut. Doses are in the range of 40 to 120 mg of the standardized extracts. Start with 40 mg per day and increase as needed.

• Pycnogenol (*Pinus pinaster*). 100 to 120 mg, 3 times per day for 3 to 12 weeks. Discontinue if relief is not experienced after 12 weeks of administration. May be combined with horse chestnut (either oral or topical) for an additive benefit.

• Selenium. Doses ranging from 50 to 1000 micrograms per day with average doses of 300 to 500 micrograms per day are suggested. In some clinical conditions, a single dose of 3000 micrograms intravenously is administered on the day of surgery followed by oral administration for 4 to 6 weeks. In some cases, maintenance doses of 100 micrograms per day are continued after the 6 week period. Only a doctor, nurse practitioner, or physician assistant can prescribe the intravenous administration of selenium.

Yoga

Performing these yoga postures in a continuous sequence (vinyasa) will provide mild to moderate aerobic exercise. The sun salutation provides aerobic and resistance training. Be careful not to overstrain your muscles during any exercise or with advanced postures since strenuous exercise can hinder lymph circulation.

Consult with your doctor prior to starting a yoga routine. Most often, compression sleeves are worn when doing yoga postures
Breathing (Appendix D): Ujjayi breath, kapalabhati
Poses (Appendix D): Mountain pose, sun salutation, triangle pose, twisting triangle pose, seated forward bend, legs up relaxation pose, relaxation pose

Mouth Sores

What are Mouth Sores?

Mouth sores are a symptom of mucositis, an inflammation of the lining of the digestive tract, and can occur in the lining of the mouth or on the lips. These painful ulcers may interfere with eating, drinking, talking, or breathing. Mucositis can lead to dehydration, poor nutritional status, and weight loss due to the difficulty or pain associated with eating. Mouth sores can also increase the risk of a serious infection. In some cases, mouth sores can be so severe that a patient's cancer treatment plan may need to be changed.

Cancer and its treatment contribute to the inflammation and ulcerative response of the mucous membranes in the mouth. Patients receiving certain chemotherapy drugs such as fluorouracil, methotrexate, etoposide, cytarabine and doxorubicin and/or radiation therapy to the head and neck are at increased risk of developing mouth sores. Certain infectious organisms such as the herpes simplex virus can also contribute to the development of mouth sores. Many of the therapies that are a part of stem cell transplant can also increase the risk for developing mouth sores.

How are Mouth Sores Treated by Conventional Medicine?

Preventative strategies are important including regular teeth brushing, mouth rinses, and dental checkups. Discontinue smoking as this may delay healing in the mouth. Oral cryotherapy and sucking on ice chips before and during chemotherapy treatments may also be recommended. Palifermin (Kepivance®) may be prescribed for certain patients undergoing bone marrow or stem cell transplants.

Mouth sores can also cause pain. Under these circumstances, treatment strategies are usually aimed at relieving pain. Topical painkillers such as mouthwashes containing lidocaine, or oral or intravenous pain medications may be prescribed.

Integrative Approaches to Mouth Sores

Integrative therapies focus on supporting the healing of the open sores in the gastrointestinal tract through supplements or homeopathy, nutrition remedies, and acupressure. The nutrition recommendations emphasize foods that soothe the gastrointestinal tract while providing adequate calories. The suggested supplements and homeopathy support the healing of the open sores. Homeopathy can be especially beneficial if you cannot tolerate liquids.

Before adding any integrative therapy to your treatment plan, speak with your doctor about the benefits and risks. A summary of risks may be found in the Introduction along with detailed instructions for the application of and considerations for each of the indicated therapies.

Integrative Medicine in Action

Patient Story
Integrative Medicine Plan for Mouth Sores:
Acupressure and Supplements.
Patient: James, a 19-year old man with rhabdomyosarcoma experiencing mouth sores during radiation and chemotherapy treatments.
Chief Complaint: James' doctor had told him and his parents about the possibility of developing mouth sores during his treatment. His doctor advised him to brush, floss, and rinse his mouth after all meals.
Treatment: After four radiation treatments, James began to notice a few ulcers in his mouth. The ulcers did not cause pain, but James and his parents were concerned the mouth sores might get worse. To prevent mouth sores from getting worse, James began supplementation with glutamine and sucked on ice chips before and after radiation and chemotherapy treatments. James also incorporated acupressure in his routine during the course of radiation treatment.
Outcome: James found that the mouth sores did not become more severe and healed more quickly than expected. He continued this regimen throughout the course of his treatment.

Chinese Medicine/Acupressure

According to Chinese medicine, mouth sores occur from either accumulated heat in the body rising to the mouth, lips, and head or from abundant heat in the local area resulting in a heat toxin. Certain cancers and their related therapies can cause heat to accumulate in the body, can impede local qi and blood circulation leading to mouth sores. Chinese medicine approaches the treatment of mouth sores by clearing heat and regulating qi and blood flow in the mouth.

Acupressure
Most frequently used (Appendix A)
HT 8, LU 10, SP 2, ST 44
Secondary points (Appendix A)
DU 14, HT 5, Kid 2, LI 2, LI 4, LU 6

Herbal Teas

Herbal teas may provide topical relief from mouth sores. Drink herbal tea at room temperature, avoiding very hot or cold temperatures as this may irritate mouth sores. Be generous with honey. Honey will coat the mouth and gastrointestinal tract, easing pain, and promoting the regeneration of cells. Instructions for tea preparation may be found in Chapter 4.

- Prepare a tea with one of the following herbs: German chamomile (*Matricaria recutita*), Holy Basil (*Ocimum tenuiflorum*), or Myrrh (*Commiphora molmol*). Seep 1 to 2 tsp of each herb in 6 to 8 ounces of warm water for 5 to 10 minutes, strain. Drink the tea throughout the day, especially when mouth sores are severe.

Homeopathy

Mixtures of homeopathic remedies (TRAUMEEL S™) or individual remedies may be helpful with mouth sores. In homeopathy, the amount of liquid required is small (about 1/8 to 1/4 ounce). Consider homeopathy if you are experiencing severe pain from mucositis and having difficulty swallowing liquids.
- Cayenne. 1 tablet (6 or 12c) 3 to 5 times per day, as needed. Discontinue once mouth sores resolve.
- **TRAUMEEL S™.** This is a mixture of homeopathic remedies. For severe mouth sores, take 1 to 2 doses of the liquid 3 to 5 times per day. As your mouth sores resolve, decrease the frequency of the remedy. This may be less effective with treatments associated with high risk of mouth sores.

Nutrition

Certain foods can irritate or worsen the pain associated with mouth sores. Avoid acidic foods (oranges, grapefruit, tomato, lemons, lime), coarse foods (nuts, crackers, raw vegetables), hot and spicy foods, and alcohol. As your sores heal, you can reintroduce these foods as tolerated. Small pieces of food, and soft or pureed textures such as soup (pureed or broth-based), milk or yogurt-based shakes,

Quick Dietary Tips

- Choose soft and smooth foods; avoid rough and coarse foods
- Experiment with various food preparation methods when cooking at home or dining out

risotto, oatmeal, egg noodles, polenta, frittatas, scrambled eggs, and baked squash will be easier to eat.

Experiment with preparing your favorite foods in new ways. For example, replace spinach salad with sautéed spinach, try applesauce instead of raw apples, scramble or fry eggs instead of boiling them. Sautéing foods in extra-virgin olive oil rather than roasting will make foods easier to swallow. Be generous with the healthy oils (extra-virgin olive oil, canola oil, flax oil, grape seed oil) as they can act as a lubricant for the gastrointestinal tract.

Food Remedies

• Include garlic in your meals as it may help reduce your risk of infection in the mouth.

• Be generous with honey. Research studies have found that the nectar (a type of honey) from the tea tree (*Camellia sinensis*) plant helps prevent radiation-induced mucositis. Swish and swallow ¾ ounce of honey 15 minutes prior to radiation therapy, then 15 minutes and 6 hours after radiation. If you are unable to find this nectar, replace with honey.

• Chew on Holy Basil (Tulsi) leaves throughout the day.

• Prepare congee soup (refer to the chapter on Nausea and Vomiting) or your favorite pureed soup. To facilitate healing of the mucosal cells, be generous with protein. Choose heavy and creamy soups rather than thin, broth-based ones. You will need the extra calories during this time.

• Juice. Juices are readily tolerated during periods of mouth sores and can provide important nutrients. Choose non-acidic fruits or vegetables for juicing such as celery, carrots, kale, berries, watermelon, and cantaloupe.

Supplements

Supplements combined with herbal mouthwashes may help reduce the risk of developing mouth sores and decrease their severity. Glutamine is a nutrition supplement that has been found in clinical trials to reduce the frequency and severity of mouth sores in individuals with cancer.

• **Glutamine** is often used to prevent and manage mouth sores especially before and during chemotherapy and stem cell transplant. The dose for glutamine is 2 grams/m^2, 2 times per day. Your medical team will provide guidance on dosing per m^2. In children the maximum is four grams per dose. Begin supplementation at the start of your chemotherapy.

You may add any of the following mouthwashes:

• German chamomile (*Matricaria recutita*). Rinsing with German chamomile has been found to be beneficial for radiation-induced mouth sores. A benefit has not been found for mouth sores caused by chemotherapy; however, variations in effectiveness may be related to the timing of the chemotherapy treatment. Swish and swallow 2 to 3 times per day.
• Herbal tea mouthwash. Combine equal portions of sage (*Salvia officinalis*), goldenseal (*Hydrastis canadensis*), and raspberry leaf (*Rubus idaeus*) into 4 to 6 ounces of warm water, seep, and strain. Swish and swallow 3 to 4 times over the course of a day. You can also spit if taste is not tolerable.
• Myrrh (*Commiphora molmol*). Swish and swallow myrrh tea 2 to 3 times per day.

Nausea & Vomiting

What are Nausea and Vomiting?

Nausea is an unpleasant sensation in the throat and stomach, which is accompanied by the urge to vomit, and vomiting is the elimination of stomach contents through the mouth. Nausea and vomiting can happen prior to receiving chemotherapy treatments (anticipatory), within minutes or hours of receiving cancer treatment (acute), or up to 5 days later (delayed).

The causes of nausea and vomiting are generally related to chemotherapy, radiation therapy, the administration of other drugs, or to the disease. The class of drug, dose, and administration schedule of chemotherapy will determine the frequency and severity of nausea and vomiting. The dose and area receiving radiation therapy will also affect the severity of nausea and vomiting. With acute nausea and vomiting related to chemotherapy, several chemicals released by cells in the body trigger nausea and vomiting. Radiation treatments to the small intestine, stomach, or brain also trigger nausea and vomiting. In advanced cancer, severe constipation or bowel obstruction from a tumor can lead to nausea or vomiting. With delayed nausea and vomiting, certain moderate and highly emetogenic (known to cause vomiting) chemotherapy drugs, like cisplatin and doxorubicin, that are given at high doses or on consecutive days can trigger nausea and vomiting days after receiving chemotherapy. Delayed vomiting is also more likely to occur if you are experiencing acute vomiting.

How are Nausea and Vomiting Treated by Conventional Medicine?

Different medications may be prescribed to prevent or treat nausea and vomiting depending on when they occur. Acute and delayed nausea may be treated with anti-nausea medications such as serotonin antagonists (ondansetron, granisetron, dolasetron), dopamine antagonists (prochlorperazine, metoclopramide, haloperidol), corticosteroids (dexamethasone), benzodiazepines (lorazepam), cannabinoids (dronabinol), benzamides (metoclopramide), butyrophenones (haloperidol), and anxiolytics (lorazepam). However, these medications may not always fully control all symptoms, especially if the nausea and vomiting are anticipatory. Uncontrolled nausea or vomiting may lead to dehydration, electrolyte abnormalities, loss of appetite and weight loss, and mental anguish. Management of nausea and vomiting can be individualized. Different medications or combinations of anti-nausea medications may be prescribed until relief is managed.

Integrative Approaches to Nausea and Vomiting

There are many integrative therapies that can be beneficial for nausea and vomiting many of which have been found to be safe and effective in clinical trials. Most often, the integrative approach relies on acupuncture for the management of nausea and vomiting. Acupuncture is clinically effective for managing most types of nausea and vomiting. **Acupuncture must be delivered by a licensed acupuncturist**. For patients who do not have access to a licensed acupuncturist, acupoints can also be stimulated by acupressure as needed which can include the use of acupressure bands. Aromatherapy may be used individually or combined with any of the touch therapies. A registered dietician or nutritionist will help ensure you are maintaining caloric intake. Supplements may be considered if your regimen is not able to entirely manage your symptoms.

For anticipatory nausea and vomiting, also refer to the chapter on Anxiety and Stress.

Before adding any integrative therapy to your treatment plan, speak with your doctor about the benefits and risks. A summary of risks may be found in the Introduction along with detailed instructions for the application of and considerations for each of the indicated therapies.

Integrative Medicine in Action

Patient Story
Integrative Medicine Plan for Nausea and Vomiting:
Acupressure/Acupuncture, Aromatherapy, and Herbal Teas.
Patient: Gloria, a 64-year old woman with ovarian cancer experiencing severe nausea and occasional vomiting.
History and Complaint: Gloria's prescribed anti-nausea medications were not sufficiently managing her nausea, and she had lost a lot of weight. Her nausea and vomiting were particularly bad on the days she received her chemotherapy treatment, and severe nausea continued for several days after each treatment.
Treatment: On her way to a routine chemotherapy visit, Gloria vomited just after arriving at the outpatient center. Feeling sick and frustrated, she decided to see a licensed acupuncturist. At the acupuncture session, the acupuncturist stimulated ST 36, PC 6, and ST 40 acupoints. Gloria found that her nausea went away within minutes. Gloria learned the corresponding acupoints, so she could apply acupressure at home. Between visits to the acupuncturist, she used acupressure as needed, applying peppermint essential oil to ST 36. She also drank ginger tea 4 to 5 times per week especially when her nausea was severe.
Outcome: Over the next two months, Gloria's nausea and vomiting became less frequent and severe. She continued seeing the acupuncturist once a week and using acupressure, aromatherapy, and herbal teas at home throughout her cancer treatment.

Aromatherapy

Aromatherapy can help for anticipatory, acute, and delayed nausea and vomiting. You can use aromatherapy alone or in combination with any integrative therapy. Experiment with different oils to determine the oil that provides the greatest relief as the right oil will vary from person to person. Once you choose the oil, have it readily available over the course of the day. Instructions for application of aromatherapy may be found in Chapter 4.

Diffusion/Direct inhalation/Reflexology: Bergamot, Ginger, Grapefruit, Lemon, Orange, Peppermint
Special Applications
• Directly apply any of the above essential oils on acupressure point PC 6 and ST 36 (Appendix A).
• In order to prevent the onset of nausea and vomiting, a compress may be applied over the skin on the stomach area using any of the above essential oils.

Chinese Medicine/Acupressure

According to Chinese medical theory, nausea arises when the qi of the stomach is being forced upward against its natural tendency to flow down. This can happen for many reasons, including cold or heat generated in the stomach, overeating, and damp accumulation.

You can use acupressure at any time nausea or vomiting occurs. For constant stimulation of the PC 6 acupoint, consider using acupressure bands. These can be used intermittingly or throughout the day.

Most frequently used (Appendix A)
PC 6, ST 36
If possible, one should apply acupressure to both sides of the body on each of the points. The effect should take a few minutes, so continue to hold the points until relief is felt.
Secondary points (Appendix A)
Ren 12, SP 4
If you are experiencing acid regurgitation, add: ST 44
If symptoms worsen with strong odors, add: ST 40

Herbal Teas

Extremely hot or cold drinks may trigger nausea or vomiting. If you prefer sweetened tea, choose honey or agave nectar. Instructions for tea preparation may be found in Chapter 4.

- Fresh Ginger root (*Zingiber officinale*). This tea can be particularly beneficial for dry heaves. Grate fresh ginger root, add 1/2 to 1 tsp of grated ginger to warm water, seep for 5 to 10 minutes (for a stronger flavor, seep longer), strain. Add one teaspoon of honey to one cup of fresh ginger tea. Drink throughout the day.
- Peppermint (*Mentha piperita*), Ginger (*Zingiber officinale*), and/or Fennel (*Foeniculum vulgare*). Seep 2 to 4 tsp of any of these herbs in 6 to 8 ounces of hot water for 5 to 10 minutes, strain. A combination of these herbs may be more effective than each individually.

Homeopathy

In most cases, the dose for treatment of nausea and vomiting is 30c (a higher potency is suggested for increased severity). Begin with a few tablets as soon as you feel nauseous, repeat the dose every 15 to 30 minutes until symptoms resolve. Once symptoms resolve, reduce the frequency of the dose to every hour or every few hours. Do not exceed 8 doses per day. For the prevention of nausea and vomiting, choose a dose of 6c potency, 1 to 2 times per day. The two remedies below are often combined.

- **Ipecacuanha.** Uncontrolled vomiting, retching that is not relieved by vomiting, sensitive to smells.
- **Nux vomica.** Nausea that feels better after vomiting, retching, triggered by food; associated with stress and anxiety.

Nutrition

Many patients find it difficult to eat anything during periods of nausea or vomiting. Eat frequent but small meals, meals at room temperature, and eliminate bothersome odors or flavors. Consume simple and bland foods. Make sure you drink enough, even if it is only small amounts at a time to avoid dehydration. Coconut water is a natural way to replace electrolytes and is preferred over sports drinks which can contain a lot of sugar.

Quick Dietary Tips

- Choose simple bland foods. Avoid foods with a strong flavor
- Rehydrate with coconut water
- Choose a protein-rich meal at least once per day

Nutrition should be combined with other integrative approaches and medications prescribed by your doctor.

Food Remedies

• Congee (Rice Porridge). Congee is easy on the stomach, readily digested, and very versatile. A typical Chinese Congee includes:

o 1 cup white rice
o 12 cups water
o 1 to 2 tsp salt

There are many different versions of congee. You can vary the consistency:

o Thick: 1 cup rice to 8 cups water
o Medium:1 cup rice to 10 cups water
o Thin: 1 cup rice to 13 cups water

If you prefer a heartier, protein-rich dish, add beans or chicken. If you favor sweet flavors, add fresh or dried fruit or agave nectar. For additional relief, add poppy seed. Cook until rice is slightly overcooked and has a soupy consistency.

• Frozen fruit slices tend to be better tolerated than fresh fruits. Suggested flavors are papaya, mango, berries, apple, or pear slices. You can purchase these ready-made or prepare them yourself. Put fresh fruit in the freezer for 15-45 minutes for an immediate food remedy for nausea and vomiting.

• Clear broth soups may be tolerated warm or at room temperature. The ingredients can vary depending on the severity of your nausea. To increase protein, add extra-firm tofu or shredded chicken or turkey. To satisfy a carbohydrate craving, add noodles (plain or egg noodles) or brown rice. For immune support, add seaweed (wakame) or any other leafy vegetable (spinach, kale, shredded Brussels sprouts).

• Fresh or dried ginger. Fresh ginger root is stronger and will provide more immediate relief. Be generous with ginger as a flavoring for any dish including cooked vegetables and meat-based entrees. One tsp of grated fresh ginger with two tsp of orange zest or peel can be added to any soup for flavoring.

• Emphasize high protein-based meals or shakes. Clinical studies have found that higher protein intake decreases chemotherapy-related nausea. High protein shakes (40 grams per meal) as meal replacements or a protein-rich diet *combined* with ginger supplements (1 gram per day) is an effective combination, particularly for delayed nausea. Follow this regimen for three days following chemotherapy for management of delayed nausea and vomiting.

• Roasted pumpkin or squash seeds. According to TCM therapy, roast seeds at 350 degrees Fahrenheit for 5 to 10 minutes and season lightly with salt. You may add a sprinkle of ginger powder on the seeds for an added benefit.

Reflexology

Reflexology may be most helpful for anticipatory and acute nausea and vomiting. Information on reflexology technique can be found in Chapter 4.

Foot Points
R: Gall bladder reflex
T: Diaphragm, esophagus, spinal, stomach reflexes

Hand Points
R: Gall bladder reflex
T: Diaphragm, esophagus, spinal, stomach reflexes

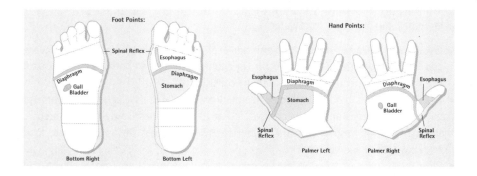

Supplements

Clinical studies suggest that ginger supplements may be effective in managing nausea and vomiting when taken for a brief time during the chemotherapy cycle that is associated with nausea or vomiting. It is not necessary to supplement with ginger during the entire course of your treatment.

• **Ginger (*Zingiber officinale*).** One gram dried ginger root per day. Begin supplementation 3 to 5 days prior to your cycle of therapy and continue for 3 to 5 days after receiving your chemotherapy or radiation.

Visual Imagery

Sit up with your back straight. If you are unable to sit up because you are not feeling well enough, lie down with pillows under your head and upper back, so your head is higher than your stomach. Close your eyes and focus on your breath. Gently listen to yourself inhale and then exhale. Repeat this five times. Once you feel relaxed, try to focus on the pain and discomfort. Pay attention to what it feels like to be nauseous. See your nausea as a color. What color is it? See your color start to change to a soft blue. Picture that soft blue light inside your stomach or wherever you feel uncomfortable. Feel that soft blue light slowly calming down the angry, sick feeling. Allow that light to fill your body. Feel your body relaxing and slowly feel the nausea start to go away. Continue this visualization as often as needed. If you feel too sick or are vomiting, wait until the nausea has lessened in intensity before following this visualization.

Repeat as needed.

Yoga

Dim all the lights and lie flat on your back or in a semi-reclining position. Begin using the breathing techniques described below. When your feelings of nausea begin to lessen, slowly sit up and come into Child's pose and then Relaxation pose. If needed, follow the restorative modifications that can be found in appendix D. Avoid posture sequences (vinyasas) that require you to move up and down from the floor.

Breathing (Appendix D): Ujjayi breath, alternate nostril breathing
Poses (Appendix D): Child's pose, relaxation pose

Pain

What is Pain?

Pain is an unpleasant, hurting sensation that is associated with tissue damage and has both physical and emotional characteristics. Pain may be categorized as acute (less than 1 to 3 months) or chronic (persistent).

Pain experienced during cancer treatment may be directly related to the cancer due to a tumor pressing on adjacent tissue or from the cancer spreading to the bone or other parts of the body. Pain may also develop as a result of side effects associated with cancer treatment such as peripheral neuropathy, radiation burns and scarring, steroid-induced joint pain, and mouth sores. Pain can also follow surgery or other cancer-related treatment procedures.

How is Pain Treated by Conventional Medicine?

Cancer pain will be carefully monitored by your medical team on a regular basis. Management strategies may include relieving the source of pain by reducing the size of the tumor through the use of cancer therapies, using pain medications, and utilizing cognitive-behavioral approaches such as relaxation, distraction, and the application of heat and cold. Mild to moderate pain can be managed with mild painkillers like acetaminophen, while moderate to severe pain is managed with opioid drugs such as morphine. Adjuvant drugs such as antidepressants, anticonvulsants, or corticosteriods may also be prescribed for difficult pain syndromes like bone pain.

Integrative Approaches to Pain

Integrative therapies can provide pain relief and block receptors that promote the sensation of pain. Most notably, in clinical studies acupuncture has been found to be safe and effective in treating cancer pain. Acupuncture can only be administered by a licensed acupuncturist. Acupressure will have milder effect, but has the advantage in that it can self-administered. Visual imagery and massage are beneficial during an acute pain crisis. Yoga, especially yogic breathing exercises, can also help alleviate all types of pain. When pain is superficial, homeopathic creams or ointments applied to the skin may be helpful when combined with either massage or reflexology.

Before adding any integrative therapy to your treatment plan, speak with your doctor about the benefits and risks. A summary of risks may be found in the Introduction along with detailed instructions for the application of and considerations for each of the indicated therapies.

Integrative Medicine in Action

Patient Story
Integrative Medicine Plan for Pain:
Acupuncture and Visual Imagery.
Patient: Betty, a 72-year old woman with advanced lung cancer.
Chief Complaint: Betty was in extreme pain due to bone metastases. Her pain was especially severe in her lower back. Despite taking morphine and receiving radiation to the spine, Betty remained uncomfortable and inconsolable.
Treatment: Betty's oncologist referred her to a licensed acupuncturist who was experienced in working with patients with cancer. Betty's family arranged for the acupuncturist to visit her at home on a twice-weekly basis. Sessions began with acupuncture using points SI 3, UB 10, UB 40, and UB 62. Her acupuncturist also led Betty through a visualization during which she imagined a magnet gently removing pain from her body.
Outcome: Betty's acupuncturist helped her find solace and support during her cancer treatment. The visual imagery helped her relax and be more physically comfortable. Betty continued to practice the visual imagery on the days she did not receive acupuncture services.

Aromatherapy

Essential oils can be applied directly on the skin with massage or reflexology. Choose the most appealing essential oil from the list below for either application. Discontinue aromatherapy if your pain increases with its application. Instructions for application of aromatherapy may be found in Chapter 4.

Muscle Pain
Bath: Basil, Cypress, Lavender, Peppermint, Sweet marjoram
Direct Application/Massage: Black pepper, Cypress, Lavender, Lemongrass, Peppermint

Nerve Pain
Bath: Lavender, Peppermint
Direct Application/Massage: Black pepper, Lavender, Peppermint

Joint and Bone Pain
Bath: Cypress, Helichrysum, Peppermint, Spruce, Wintergreen
Direct Application/Massage: Black pepper, Cypress, Helichrysum, Peppermint

Chinese Medicine/Acupressure

The diagnosis of pain from a Chinese medicine approach will depend on the location and quality of the pain. Pain occurs when there is a disruption or blockage in the flow of qi and blood through an area and can be a result of a variety of factors. For example, an invasion of wind, cold, and damp from the environment into the muscles is a common cause of pain. This pain will be worse in damp, cold weather and will feel better with the application of heat. Pain can also arise when the body is weak from chronic illness and the muscles are not properly nourished. This type of pain will feel dull and achy and will improve with rest. Acupressure can help regulate the flow of qi and blood in the body; therefore, it can be an effective way to manage all types of pain. Acupuncture is used for a deeper effect.

Acupressure
Acupressure should be applied to the tight, tender points in the area of discomfort. Press points above and below the pain. If the painful area is red, swollen, inflamed, or site of the tumor, avoid it and press on the muscle around the redness. If there is swelling, apply acupressure around the area, but not directly on it.

Most frequently used (Appendix A)
GB 34, LI 4, SP 21
If pain comes and goes and moves from joint to joint, especially in the wrists, elbow, knees, and ankles with a limited range of motion, add: GB 20, SJ 6, SP 10
If pain is severe and stabbing and is alleviated by warmth and aggravated by cold, add: DU 4, Kid 7, Ren 4, UB 23. A warm, moist compress to the affected area can also provide relief for pain.
If pain is accompanied by soreness, swelling, stiffness, and heaviness in the muscles and joints which is worse on humid rainy days, add: SP 6, SP 9, ST 40

Homeopathy

Application of homeopathic creams or ointments to the skin may help relieve both chronic and acute pain especially when combined with massage or reflexology. Apply the topical remedies as needed.

• **Arnica or Capsaicin.** Apply Arnica or Capsaicin directly over the area of pain and massage into the skin. Capsaicin is especially good for nerve pain whereas Arnica is better for muscle-type pain.

Massage

Massage may help with both acute and chronic pain. Receiving a massage by a caregiver will allow you to relax and focus on the release of pain. Practicing visualization during your massage can enhance the benefits. Use any of the three techniques mentioned in the Introduction as long as the area of pain is not red, swollen, inflamed, or the site of a tumor. Self massage is not optimal for pain management. Information on the recommended massage techniques may be found in Chapter 4.

Massage by a Caregiver

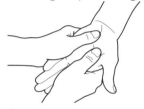

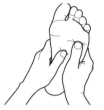

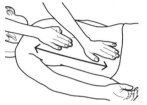

1 Start by massaging the hands using circular petrissage motions. This will initiate the relaxation process.

2 Massage the feet with general petrissage grasping and small stroke technique.

3 Move to the back of the person and have them lay on their belly. Massage the entire back starting from the upper back and moving down to the lower back with long effleurage strokes. Return the person to lying on their back.

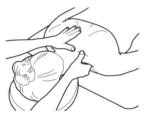

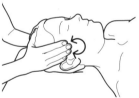

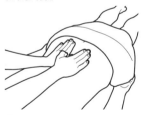

4 Massage the back of the neck and shoulder area on the upper trapezius muscle with short petrissage motions, using small strokes, circular, and pinching technique.

5 Using small circular petrissage motions, massage the temples.

6 Finish the massage by massaging the local area of pain with any of the three techniques depending on how big the area. For example, use friction technique for a small area and use effleurage and petrissage for a larger area.

Nutrition

Dietary change is not recommended for acute pain conditions, but may help to manage chronic pain by augmenting the effects of many prescribed medications.

An anti-inflammatory diet is a dietary plan frequently promoted for chronic pain. The anti-inflammatory diet is low in compounds that stimulate the cascade of biochemical events leading to inflammation thereby preventing inflammation from occurring. This mechanism is similar to that of aspirin. The clinical benefits are not immediate. The diet must be adopted as part of a lifestyle approach to experience the benefits.

There are many variations of the anti-inflammatory diet, but it is most similar in structure to the Mediterranean diet. Although the anti-inflammatory diet has not been scientifically evaluated in any formalized manner, observational studies have found that the Mediterranean diet is associated with decreased inflammation, and with reductions in heart disease, autoimmune disorders, and cancer.

Adopting an anti-inflammatory diet can be challenging. The anti-inflammatory diet is less about excluding foods and more about choosing the right foods. The anti-inflammatory diet emphasizes lean proteins (poultry, fish, beans), fruits and vegetables, whole grains (brown rice, kashi), healthy fats (olive oil, fatty fish, nuts, seeds, avocado), and select spices (turmeric, cumin, curry, garlic, ginger, cinnamon). Variations on the anti-inflammatory diet may limit or restrict intake of gluten, dairy, or other food allergens. Avoidance of these nutrients is only useful if you have food allergies or sensitivities. Work with your doctor or nutritionist to determine if exclusion of these foods could be beneficial for you. A summary of daily dietary goals of the anti-inflammatory diet is included in this chapter.

Many of the foods integral to the anti-inflammatory diet are not a component of the standard Western diet, so patience, an open mind, and a willingness to experiment with new foods are critical to its success. Cooking and eating only the freshest foods is the foundation of this diet. Strive for eating fresh foods at least two times per day. During periods of extreme fatigue, purchasing ready-made fresh foods can be an alternative. To ease the transition, create a weekly shopping list and meal plan. A sample shopping menu is included in this chapter. This will help you become familiar with any new foods and reduce the pressure of last minute menu planning. Examples of simple substitutions and shopping lists are provided below. *Begin with simple and comfortable changes and move towards more complex ones.*

For example:
- *Instead of* peanut butter *Choose* almond or cashew butter
- *Instead of* turkey and mayonnaise sandwich *Choose* turkey with avocado or any bean-based spread
- *Instead of* white rice *Choose* brown rice or quinoa
- *Instead of* tuna salad *Choose* salmon salad
- *Instead of* coffee *Choose* white or green tea
- *Instead of* high-sugar breakfast cereal *Choose* a high fiber, Omega-3 enriched cereal

- *Instead* of a hamburger *Choose* a turkey or vegetable burger with sautéed onions with sweet potato fries or any fruit or vegetable of your choice
- *Instead* of Caesar salad *Choose* grilled chicken salad with olive oil-based vinaigrette
- *Instead* of pork-fried rice *Choose* vegetable-fried rice
- *Instead* of Ham or breaded cutlets *Choose* vegetables, grilled/baked chicken or turkey
- *Instead* of ice cream *Choose* gelato or sorbet
- Instead of white bread *Choose* 100% whole wheat or multi grain varieties
- *Instead* of eggs *Choose* eggs fortified with omega 3

Anti-Inflammatory Grocery List

Protein

- Fresh or canned wild salmon
- Sardines
- Chicken or Turkey
- Omega 3 fortified eggs
- Beans of your choice

Grains

- **Breakfast Cereal:** Any cereal fortified with Omega 3's and having at least 4 to 5 grams of fiber per serving
- **Grains/Pasta:** Brown rice, quinoa, couscous, orzo, or kashi

Fruits/Vegetables/Snacks

- **3 to 5 dark colored vegetables:** Broccoli, Brussels sprouts, squash, mesclun, lettuce, kale, carrots, bok choy, sweet potatoes, string beans, onions (all varieties), and peppers
- Tart or sour cherries (these are not the same as sweet cherries)
- **Mushrooms:** Shitaki, maitaki, reishi
- **Nuts or Nut Bars (avoid high fructose corn syrup):** Almonds, cashews, pistachios
- **3 to 5 different colored fruits:** Avocado, berries, oranges, grapes, melon/cantaloupe
- Granola

Condiments/Oils

- **Spices:** Cinnamon, curry, cumin, garlic, parsley, oregano, mint, rosemary, ginger, chili peppers, basil
- **Oils:** Use extra virgin olive oil for sautéing foods; experiment with flax, grapeseed, or walnut oil for salad dressing (these oils are not for cooking)
- A favorite bean variety or bean spreads (hummus, white bean dip)

Daily Dietary Goals
The Anti-Inflammatory Diet

	Goal	Choose	Avoid
Carbohydrates	Choose a whole grain product 4 to 5 times per week Consume 25 to 30 grams of fiber per day All cereal should have at least 4 to 5 grams of fiber per serving	Whole-grains (quinoa, brown rice, kashi, whole wheat couscous) High fiber breakfast cereals, any fruits or vegetables, nuts and seeds, whole-grain products 100% whole wheat bread Pasta: Cook al dente. Use olive oil-based sauces	White flour-based grains (e.g. white rice, white bread, pasta), grains served with heavy sauces (e.g. fettuccini alfredo) Sugar-based cereals or any cereal with less than 4 to 5 grams of fiber per serving Cream-based sauces
Protein	Eat 1 to 2 daily portions of the recommended sources of lean protein	Lean beef, poultry, cage-free eggs, beans, yogurt	Beef, pork, breaded or fried animal products, processed deli meats, fast food sandwiches/burgers
Fats (Oils/Condiments)	Eat a daily portion of some type of healthy fat	Olive oil, canola oil, vegetable-based mayonnaise, avocado and bean spreads, coconut milk	Butter, vegetable oil, shortening, hydrogenated fats, high-fat dairy products

(Continued)

(Continued)

	Goal	Choose	Avoid
Fruits/ Vegetables	2 to 3 different fruits and 2 to 3 different vegetables each day	Choose fresh over frozen or canned	Canned or packaged fruits with added sugar, fruit juices, fried vegetables
Snacks	Snack wisely, only snack on those foods with some health benefits	Grain/nut bars, nuts (almonds, cashews, walnuts), any fruit or vegetable, dried beans Sorbet, gelato, yogurt	Peanuts, processed snacks (cookies, snack breads, cakes), foods with high-fructose corn syrup
Beverages	All daily drinks should be in the "green" category	Water, as needed White and green tea, sparkling water (non-sweetened), fresh green juices	Soda, caffeinated power drinks, any beverage with high-fructose corn syrup
Spices	Add beneficial spices to every meal	Ginger, garlic, turmeric, cumin, curry, cinnamon, basil, mint, rosemary	Heavily salted foods

Reflexology

The site of pain is often too tender to touch. Reflexology is a way to manage pain without aggravating the affected area. If pain is on the hands or feet, avoid reflexology and choose another integrative therapy. Information on reflexology technique can be found in Chapter 4.

Foot Points
R: Adrenal reflexes
T: Diaphragm, solar plexus, spinal reflexes; lateral line of foot, neck/shoulder line, corresponding reflexes. For example, if you are experiencing shoulder pain, use the shoulder reflex or if you have knee pain use the knee reflex. Refer to full foot chart in the Appendix.

Hand Points
R: Adrenal reflexes
T: Diaphragm, spinal reflexes; neck/shoulder line, corresponding reflexes. For example, if you are experiencing shoulder pain, use the shoulder reflex or if you have knee pain use the knee reflex. Refer to full hand chart in the Appendix.

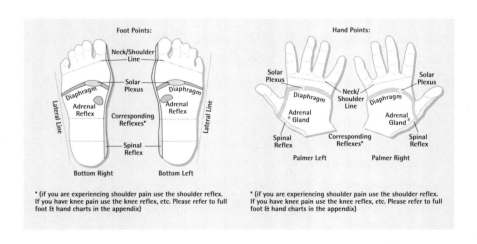

* (if you are experiencing shoulder pain use the shoulder reflex. If you have knee pain use the knee reflex, etc. Please refer to full foot & hand charts in the appendix)

* (if you are experiencing shoulder pain use the shoulder reflex. If you have knee pain use the knee reflex, etc. Please refer to full foot & hand charts in the appendix)

Visual Imagery

Make yourself comfortable by lying down or sitting in a chair with your spine straight. Put yourself in a position that causes the least amount of pain. Close your eyes and focus on your breath. If the area of pain takes your focus away from your breath, just gently refocus. Keep this up until all of your attention is on your breath. The breath should be normal, not forced or held.

When you feel you have sufficiently put all your attention on your breath, bring your attention to the area of pain. Imagine a magnetic force or a giant magnet (whatever works for you) hovering over the area of pain. Imagine this magnet pulling all the painful energy into itself. See it pulling the pain away from your body, your leg, your arm, your chest, your head, wherever the pain may be. Imagine your body easily letting go of the pain and sending it into this magnetic force. Stay with this image for as long as it takes.

This magnet is pulling all your pain away. Now imagine this magnetic force or giant magnet drift away and disappear. This magnetic force is holding all the pain it has pulled away from you. Go back to the breath and stay with this focus, relaxing your whole body. At your own pace, open your eyes and come back into your space.

Repeat as often as necessary.

Yoga

Yoga manages the emotional and physical aspects of pain. Yoga postures and breathing exercises allow you to bring consciousness to the process of breathing which are helpful with coping with both acute and chronic pain. Sun salutation is meditation in motion and keeps your focus away from the pain. For the prevention of musculoskeletal pain, practice sun salutations daily.

Breathing (Appendix D): Ujjayi breath, alternate nostril breathing
Poses (Appendix D): Sun salutation, legs up relaxation pose, child's pose, relaxation pose

Peripheral Neuropathy

What is Peripheral Neuropathy?

Peripheral neuropathy is the inflammation, injury, or deterioration of the sensory or motor peripheral nerve fibers, which are located outside of the brain and spinal cord. Peripheral sensory nerve fibers carry information to the brain for interpretation, whereas peripheral motor nerve fibers are responsible for maintaining muscle tone.

Cancer-related peripheral neuropathy is often the result of injury to the peripheral nerves due to chemotherapy, radiation therapy, or tumor. Several chemotherapy drugs increase the risk of developing peripheral neuropathy, the most common being vinca alkaloid chemotherapeutic agents which include vincristine, vinorelbine, and vinblastine. Other chemotherapy drugs such as cisplatin, carboplatin, docetaxel, paclitaxel, bortezomib, and thalidomide can also cause damage to peripheral nerves.

Sensory neuropathy usually affects the sense of touch and feeling in the nerves in the hands and feet. A feeling of tingling, burning, or numbness is commonly described and may worsen with touch. With motor neuropathy, patients may have difficulty walking and moving around. Balance and coordination problems may develop, or there may be difficulties with everyday tasks such as brushing teeth or buttoning clothes. Muscle cramping or muscle loss in the hands and feet may also develop.

How is Peripheral Neuropathy Treated by Conventional Medicine?

Medications may be prescribed to manage the pain and discomfort associated with peripheral neuropathy. Medications include tricyclic antidepressants such as amitriptyline (Elavil®) or other antidepressants belonging to the class of selective serotonin and norepinephrine reuptake inhibitors such as duloxetine (Cymbalta®). Anticonvulsant medications including gabapentin (Neurontin®) or pregabalin (Lyrica®) may also be prescribed. Pain may be managed with nonsteroidal anti-inflammatory drugs or long-acting opioid pain medications. Topical medications such as the Lidocaine patch 5% (Lidoderm®) may also help.

Non-prescription recommendations may include regular exercise or transcutaneous electrical nerve stimulation (TENS).

Integrative Approaches to Peripheral Neuropathy

The prevention or treatment of neuropathy will determine the integrative therapy best indicated. For prevention, speak with your doctor about supplementing with glutamine. Glutamine may prevent the development or progression of early signs of neuropathy. For patients with moderate to severe neuropathy, touch therapies, especially if combined with aromatherapy may be beneficial. Topical supplements may help with pain associated with both sensory and motor neuropathy. Yoga can be especially beneficial for management of motor neuropathy.

Before adding any integrative therapy to your treatment plan, speak with your doctor about the benefits and risks. A summary of risks may be found in the Introduction along with detailed instructions for the application of and considerations for each of the indicated therapies.

Integrative Medicine in Action

Patient Story
Integrative Medicine Plan for Peripheral Neuropathy:
Homeopathy, Reflexology, and Yoga.
Patient: Juan, a 43-year old man diagnosed with Non-Hodgkin Lymphoma experiencing moderate peripheral neuropathy after receiving three doses of vincristine.
Chief Complaint: Each week Juan found the tingling and numbness in his fingertips, feet, and toes were getting worse. He had trouble walking and would occasionally lose his balance. If he dropped a small object like a coin or pen, he had a hard time picking it up.
Treatment: Juan's son used capsaicin cream with a reflexology technique to the tips of the fingers and toes. To help manage his motor neuropathy, Juan began a daily yoga sequence which focused on improving movement, coordination, and balance.
Outcome: After a few weeks, Juan was able to walk with better balance and could pick up small objects again. Although his peripheral neuropathy was not completely resolved, he felt more comfortable and confident about resuming his normal daily activities.

Aromatherapy

Choose an appealing scent from the suggested oils and combine it with any of the touch therapies, but do not combine with creams or ointments applied to the skin such as capsaicin cream. Consider daily foot baths to help bring circulation to your feet. Instructions for application of aromatherapy may be found in Chapter 4.

Compress/Direct Application/Foot Bath/Massage/Reflexology: Clove, Lemongrass, Peppermint.

Chinese Medicine/Acupressure

When the qi and blood in the channels are obstructed and cannot reach an area, feelings of numbness and weakness can occur. Chinese medicine approaches neuropathy by promoting qi and blood flow through the affected area. Acupressure points are selected based on the location of the neuropathy.

Acupressure
Most frequently used (Appendix A)
For neuropathy located on the lower limb: GB 34, GB 40, Liv 3, SP 5, ST 31, ST 41, and all Ba Feng points. Apply acupressure along the lower Gallbladder channel which is a straight line that begins at GB 34 and ends at GB 40.
For neuropathy located on the upper limb: LI 4, LI 5, LI 10, LI 15, SI 5, SJ 4, and all Ba Xie points. Apply acupressure along the lower San Jiao channel which is a straight line that begins at SJ 9 and ends at SJ 4.

Homeopathy

Topical administration of homeopathic gels or creams may help relieve pain associated with neuropathy. Be careful not to apply the gel or cream into any open wounds, eyes, nasal, or any other open areas. Do not combine with aromatherapy.

• Capsaicin ointment or cream. Use gentle massage and apply the capsaicin gel or ointment over the area experiencing neuropathic pain. Administer this treatment 1 to 2 times per day or as needed. Discontinue treatment once relief is obtained.

Massage

For all types of neuropathy, only use massage with light pressure. You can combine massage with aromatherapy or any topical remedies. Information on the recommended massage techniques may be found in Chapter 4.

Massage by a Caregiver

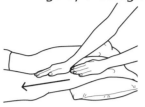
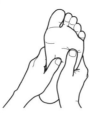
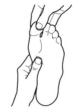

1 Massage one limb starting with long strokes in an upward direction from the ankle to the knee.

2 Repeat on the other limb.

3 Massage the feet using grasping, circular, sweeping petrissage motion.

4 Using friction technique, use small strokes on each toe one at a time.

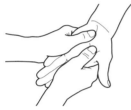
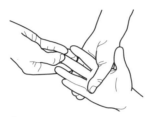

5 Massage the hands, one at a time, using grasping and circular motions on palms and backs of hands.

6 Using small stroke friction technique, massage each finger separately.

Self Massage

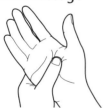
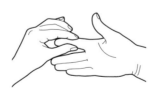
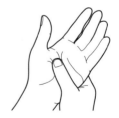

1 Apply a small amount of body lotion on your hands. With your left hand, massage the right palm using circular petrissage motions.

2 Grasp each finger from the base and squeeze up to the tip. Repeat this on all fingers.

3 With your right hand, repeat the sequence on the left palm and fingers. Gently pinch each fingertip.

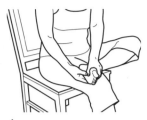 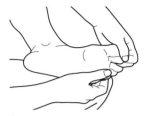

4 If you can reach your own feet, massage the whole foot with petrissage motions.

5 Grasp each toe and squeeze from the base to the tips.

6 Gently pinch the tips of each toe. Repeat this sequence two times per day until feeling comes back.

Reflexology

For all types of neuropathy, only apply gentle pressure. If you are experiencing peripheral neuropathy, reflexology applied to the whole foot or hand is indicated. If your neuropathy is too painful to touch, apply reflexology to the unaffected area. For example, if your hands are too sensitive, apply reflexology to the foot points described below. Information on reflexology technique can be found in Chapter 4.

Foot Points
F: Brain reflex on all the tips of the toes
H: Pituitary reflexes
T: Diaphragm, hypothalamus, sciatic, spinal reflexes; neck/shoulder line, waist and heel line

Hand Points
F: Brain reflex on all the tips of the fingers
H: Pituitary reflexes
T: Diaphragm, spinal reflexes; whole thumb

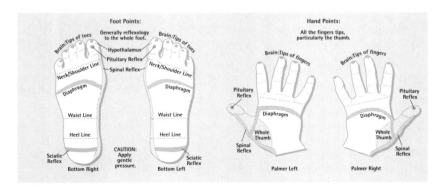

Supplements

Glutamine is a nutrition supplement that is often used in patients undergoing cancer treatment and has a wide safety profile. Glutamine may help to prevent sensory and motor neuropathy; however, it is not useful if you are experiencing severe or debilitating neuropathy. Supplement with glutamine at the beginning and throughout your chemotherapy cycle associated with peripheral neuropathy. If you begin to develop severe neuropathy that is not relieved with glutamine within a 3 to 4 week time frame, discontinue supplementation.

- **Glutamine.** Adult dose: 10 grams, three times per day; Pediatric dose: 6 grams/m^2, 2 times per day. Consult with your medical team for guidance on dosing per m^2. Begin supplementation the day after the first dose of chemotherapy associated with neuropathy. If no improvements are observed within a 3 to 4 week time period, discontinue supplementation.

Yoga

Standing postures can improve balance and coordination and may help you perform daily activities. The selected yoga sequence aims to restore balance and coordination. Backbends are included for their benefit to the nervous system. Begin with sun salutation, chair pose, cobra pose, and cobbler's pose. Add additional poses after you master this initial sequence. If you experience any pain during yoga practice, come to rest in relaxation pose.

Breathing (Appendix D): Ujjyai breath, alternate nostril breathing
Poses for motor peripheral neuropathy (Appendix D): Sun salutation, mountain pose, chair pose (without raising your arms over your head), tree pose, standing head to knee pose, dancer's pose, triangle pose, straight leg seated spinal twist, cobra pose, bow pose, camel pose, cobbler's pose, relaxation pose

Radiation Burns

What are Radiation Burns?

A radiation burn is redness or a sunburn-like appearance that develops on the skin in any area of the body receiving radiation treatment. Radiation treatment causes skin cells to break down in the area being irradiated, and when radiation treatments are frequent, skin cells do not have enough time to grow back, causing the redness to linger. Radiation burns may develop a few weeks after beginning radiation treatment. Although the redness generally goes away shortly after completing all radiation treatments, in some cases, the skin will continue to look darker.

How are Radiation Burns Treated by Conventional Medicine?

Good skin care can reduce the redness associated with radiation burns. These practices include not rubbing the area, using only lukewarm water on the area, wearing loose fitting clothes made of soft fabrics, and protecting your skin from sun exposure. Doctors may recommend cleaning the radiation area with mild, unscented soap as a preventive measure, and if burns develop, may also suggest using an absorbent, topical, and non-alcohol based ointment and monitoring for any skin irritations.

Integrative Approaches to Radiation Burns

The goal of integrative medicine for radiation burns is to relieve pain and burning sensations of the skin. The suggested therapies will not prevent the burns from occurring, but they can help minimize the pain associated with the burn and support healing in the area. Review the topical remedies with your radiation oncologist. Do not apply topical agents just before receiving radiation treatment. Only apply topical therapies **after** receiving radiation therapy and do not apply over open wounds.

Before adding any integrative therapy to your treatment plan, speak with your doctor about the benefits and risks. A summary of risks may be found in the Introduction along with detailed instructions for the application of and considerations for each of the indicated therapies.

Integrative Medicine in Action

Patient Story
Integrative Medicine Plan for Radiation Burns:
Topical Supplements (creams or ointments applied to skin).
Patient: Wendy, a 33-year old woman with nasopharyngeal carcinoma experiencing severe radiation burns.
Chief Complaint: Following three weeks of daily radiation treatments to the head and neck, Wendy developed radiation burns that became so dark and prominent that she became withdrawn and did not want to see any friends and family.
Treatment: After looking for information on the Internet, Wendy decided to consult with an herbalist to see if there were any alternative options for treating her radiation burns. The herbalist instructed her on the use of topical supplements after receiving radiation. Wendy applied aloe vera three to five times daily to soothe the burn.
Outcome: Wendy's skin discoloration began to lighten while using this topical supplement, and she began feeling comfortable enough to engage with her family and friends again.

Aromatherapy

Essential oils can be soothing and cooling to the skin. Essential oils can be added to an aloe vera mist, or applied individually. If diluting essential oils in a carrier oil, use oils that are 100% alcohol free. Instructions for application of aromatherapy may be found in Chapter 4.

Bath/Compress/Cosmetics Addition: Frankincense, Helichrysum, Lavender
Direct Application: Lavender
Special Applications
• Add 15 to 20 drops of Lavender to 1/2 ounce of aloe in a mister bottle. Shake vigorously before use and spray on skin.

Homeopathy

Homeopathic ointments or creams may provide relief of burns associated with radiation therapy. Apply the cream or ointment *after* receiving radiation therapy, as needed. **Do not apply any creams or ointments prior to receiving radiation treatment.**

• **Calendula cream or ointment.** Apply to the affected area as needed.
• Urtica urens. Apply to affected area as needed.

Supplements

Apply the suggested remedies after treatment to soothe burning and support skin regeneration. Prior to your next radiation treatment, clean the area using the skin care guidelines provided by your radiation oncologist.

• Aloe vera. Apply topically. Use pure aloe vera gel or the gel found in the leaves of the aloe vera plant as this is different than aloe vera juice. Aloe plants can be found at many health food stores or a plant nursery. To extract the gel, slice down the seam of the leaf, being careful not to slice the interior portion of the leaf. Open the leaf as if you were opening a book. The middle will be filled with a gel-like substance, and the gummy part will be found along the interior side of the leaf. Rub the leaf over the exposed area, being careful to apply the gummy part directly to the affected area. Use a fresh leaf for each application. Apply 3 to 5 times per day or as needed.
• Sea vegetables. Kombu is a sea vegetable that can be found in most health food stores and is sold as long pieces. Soak individual kombu pieces in a bowl of cold water and apply directly to the burned area for 10 to 15 minutes. Apply 3 to 5 times per day or as needed.
• Tofu. Slice soft to firm tofu and place on the affected area. Apply for approximately 10 minutes or until relief is experienced. Apply 3 to 5 times per day or as needed.
• Vitamin E oil. Apply to the affected area 3 to 5 times per day.

Visual Imagery

Sit or lie down comfortably. Close your eyes and focus on your breath. As you breathe in, imagine your body being filled up with cooling, healing energy. As you breathe out, imagine all pains, aches, tensions, and feelings of discomfort leave with the breath. Breathe in the healing, cooling energy, breathe out all tension. Repeat five times.

Feel the area that has been radiated. What is that area telling you? Is it hot? Is it painful? Is it numb or tingling? Once you focus on the area and what it's telling you, imagine a cool deep blue light filling up the area. Feel the light bringing relaxation and a cooling sensation. Imagine it replacing all tension and heat with coolness, as if a cool breeze covers the area. Stay with this image until you feel any change in sensation of the affected area.

When you feel you have a clear image of the cooling blue light, at your own pace, open your eyes.

This is a step-by-step process. Tell yourself that every day you practice this visualization, the skin of the radiated area becomes more and more relaxed, cooled, and healed. Repeat daily.

Shortness of Breath

What is Shortness of Breath?

Shortness of breath, or dyspnea, is the condition of breathlessness. Shortness of breath is often described as a smothering feeling, tightness in the chest, or inability to get enough air. Shortness of breath may be temporary (acute), persistent (chronic), or occur at rest or with exertion.

Cancer, cancer treatments, and other medical and psychological conditions can contribute to shortness of breath. Shortness of breath is generally caused by lung cancer or a tumor that has spread from another organ to the lungs. Some other common causes of shortness of breath include decreased lung capacity following surgery to the lungs; radiation pneumonitis following the completion of radiation therapy; low red blood cell count (anemia) from chemotherapy or radiation therapy; toxicity to the lungs from chemotherapy agents such as bleomycin; infection; anxiety and stress; uncontrolled pain; fluid collection in the lungs related to heart failure; other medical conditions such as obesity or asthma; and hot weather.

How is Shortness of Breath Treated by Conventional Medicine?

Management of shortness of breath is guided by relieving the underlying problem. If cancer is the principal cause of shortness of breath, chemotherapy, radiation therapy, or surgery may be necessary. Other medical interventions for shortness of breath include corticosteroids to relieve lung toxicity associated with radiation therapy or chemotherapy, discontinuation of intravenous fluid support and diuretic therapy; blood transfusions for anemia; antibiotics for pneumonia, and bronchodilators for asthma. In severe cases of shortness of breath, opioids, such as morphine, may be prescribed. Benzodiazepine medications may be suggested when shortness of breath is linked to anxiety.

Integrative Approaches to Shortness of Breath

Integrative therapies work to open up the chest and expand the breath. In our practice, yoga and visualization are often combined to assist patients in mastering deep breathing. Yoga can strengthen respiratory capacity while visualization aids in the imagination of controlled and deep breath work. Acupressure and massage can open the lung cavity directly while reflexology can help promote relaxation. Together, these therapies allow for enhanced deep breathing.

Before adding any integrative therapy to your treatment plan, speak with your doctor about the benefits and risks. A summary of risks may be found in the Introduction along with detailed instructions for the application of and considerations for each of the indicated therapies.

Integrative Medicine in Action

Patient Story
Integrative Medicine Plan for Shortness of Breath:
Acupressure, Massage, and Yoga.
Patient: Gail, a 53-year old woman with cervical cancer experiencing shortness of breath.
Chief Complaint: With fluid building up in her lungs and chest, Gail found it difficult to breathe, especially when lying down. Gail found herself physically exhausted throughout the day.
Treatment: Gail began to incorporate different yoga and acupressure techniques she discovered after reading one of her sister's complementary medicine books. Every morning Gail practiced Ujjayi breathing, followed by stimulation of the acupressure points LU 1, ST 40, and UB 23. After two weeks she added mountain pose, cobra pose, and fish pose to her regimen. Three nights per week, Gail's sister massaged her while she sat up to relieve some of the pressure from the fluid build-up in her lungs. The massage focused on the intercostal spaces, the pectoralis major muscle, the upper back, and the neck and shoulders.
Outcome: Gail was more able to breathe more freely, and attend to her daily activities.

Chinese Medicine/Acupressure

The primary organs involved in breathing are the lungs and the kidneys. The lungs function to regulate the intake and release of air thereby helping to form qi, while the kidneys serve to "grasp the qi" and hold it down. When the lungs are healthy, they fill with air, descend it downward, and fully exhale. The kidneys are able to take hold of the air, pulling it downward for a complete inhalation. If shortness of breath is due to a disruption in the flow of lung qi, there will be difficulty with exhalation; if the problem involves the kidney qi, there will be difficulty with inhalation. If the qi of both organs are affected, inhalation and exhalation may be difficult. Causes of shortness of breath may involve the buildup of cold or heat. For example, if cold has accumulated in the lungs, the shortness of breath will worsen with exposure to cold. A similar effect will occur with heat. A buildup of mucus in the lungs can also cause difficulty breathing. In this case, the shortness of breath will usually worsen when lying down.

Acupressure
Most frequently used (Appendix A)
Ding chuan, LU 1, PC 6, Ren 17, UB 13

If worse with exertion, add: Kid 6, Kid 27, LU 9, ST 36
If worse when lying down, add: LU 6, PC 5, SP 9, ST 40

If more difficult to breath in, add: Kid 3, Kid 27, UB 23
If more difficult to breath out, add: LU 7, LU 9
If accompanied by anxiety, add: HT 7, PC 7

Massage

The massage techniques presented below focus on opening up the lung cavity by relaxing the diaphragm and the muscles between the ribs. Opening the cavity gives the lungs more space to expand and contract. Information on the recommended massage techniques may be found in Chapter 4.

Massage by a Caregiver

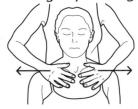 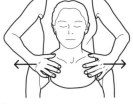 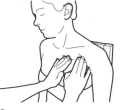

1 Stand behind the patient while they are sitting on a chair. Reach around to the chest and press your fingers against the sternum or breastbone on the midline of the chest above the breasts.

2 Pull or rake your ngers away from one another while pressing against the intercostal muscles between the ribs. Your fingers will end up by the front of the shoulders. Repeat this 3–4 times covering the whole area between the breasts and the collar bones.

3 Massage the pectoralis major muscle using a petrissage circular motion.

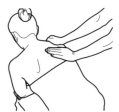 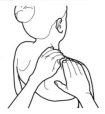

4 If the patient can lean forward, massage the upper back over the trapezius and rhomboid muscles using small petrissage circular technique in between shoulder blades.

5 Finish by using a petrissage grasping technique on the trapezius muscle of the neck and shoulder area.

Self Massage

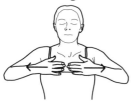 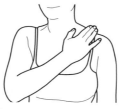 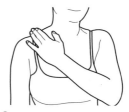

1 Press your fingertips against your sternum or breastbone just above the breasts. Pull or rake your fingers moving in an outward direction heading toward your shoulders. Repeat this process on the entire chest.

2 Take the palm of your right hand and place it against pectoralis major muscle just in front of the left shoulder. Massage the area with small circular petrissage motions.

3 Take the palm of your left hand and repeat the massage in front of the right shoulder.

4 Repeat several times a day as needed.

Reflexology

The reflexology points allow the chest and lung area to be worked on without touching the area directly. The finger walking technique across the diaphragm line helps open and relax the muscle so breaths can be deep and full. Information on reflexology technique can be found in Chapter 4.

Foot Points
T: Diaphragm, lung/chest, spinal reflexes (with focus on thoracic and cervical vertebrae reflexes); bronchial line, neck/shoulder line

Hand Points
T: Diaphragm, lung/chest, spinal reflexes

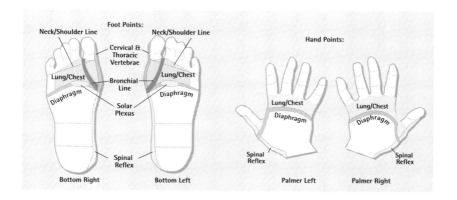

Visual Imagery

Sit up in a chair or in a place where you can keep your spine straight, or lie down on your back if you are incapable of sitting up. Close your eyes and follow your breath. Try to bring your focus to your breath. When you find your mind wandering, bring your attention back to your breath. Notice how much you can inhale without forcing. Now notice how much you can exhale without forcing. Stay with this for at least ten breaths. You are simply observing your breath. You are not doing anything but breathing.

Now feel your shoulders relaxing. Feel your upper back relaxing with every breath. Feel your muscles getting softer in between your shoulder blades (scapula). Now feel your muscles relaxing in your chest area. As you feel your muscles relax in the front and back of your upper body, notice how your inhalation reaches a little bit more deeply into your belly and your exhalation gets a little longer. Tell yourself your breathing is effortless. There is no struggle. Tell yourself the muscles in your chest and upper back area are so relaxed that more air can fill your lungs.

Now imagine your belly relaxing. Do not hold any muscle tight. Let the belly relax. Let your lower back muscles relax. Tell yourself the area from your chest to pelvis is relaxed.

Feel the inhalation going all the way down to your belly so your belly pushes out as you inhale. Feel a long, long exhalation.

Stay with this visualization for several minutes. If you cannot get the image at first, stay with it. Know that your body is relaxed and your breath is getting bigger and deeper. Notice that your breathing is more open. You can inhale, catch your breath, and exhale. Stay with this for at least 20 breaths. Do not force anything. Allow the breath to flow easily and effortlessly, easily and effortlessly. No forcing. No tightness. Let the breath flow. Visualize your lungs expanding. They are opening more and more like a balloon filled with air. They can now hold more air. Notice every breath you take relaxes you more so you can breathe more easily. Stay with this image for several minutes. When you feel you have filled your body with air, allow your focus to slowly come back into the room.

Repeat 2 to 3 times daily as needed.

Yoga

When we breathe, we typically use shallow breaths. For shortness of breath, the help of a caregiver can be especially beneficial. In this setting, the caregiver is similar to a metronome, a device that keeps the beat for a musician. The caregiver will maintain the rhythmic ujjavi breathing technique throughout the entire breathing exercise even during periods of short frantic, breaths. Below is a rhythmic breath work sequence in which the caregiver takes the lead and maintains the ebb and flow of the breath for the patient.

Partner Breathing Sequence for the Caregiver (Appendix D): Ujjayi breath.

1. Begin by sitting next to the friend or family member
2. The caregiver begins ujjavi breathing
3. Encourage the friend or family member to breath along with you using the ujjavi breath
4. The friend or family member should try to replicate the breaths of the caregiver. Do not worry if they cannot hold the rhythm, continue breathing and encourage them to join the rhythm of the ujjavi breath
5. Continue this exercise for at least ten minutes and up to three times a day

Poses (Appendix D): Mountain pose, cobra pose, camel pose, bridge pose, wheel pose, fish pose, relaxation pose

Urinary Retention and Incontinence

What are Urinary Retention and Urinary Incontinence?

Urinary retention is the when urine is not completely emptied and is abnormally kept in the bladder. Urinary incontinence, on the other hand, is the involuntary loss of urine. Types of urinary incontinence include: stress incontinence (when urine is lost during activities that increase abdominal pressure such as walking, sneezing, and coughing), urge incontinence (an overactive bladder with an uncontrollable urge to urinate but inability to reach the bathroom in time), overflow incontinence (a constant dribbling of urine), and mixed incontinence (a combination of stress and urge incontinence). Urinary retention and urinary incontinence can be temporary (acute) or persistent (chronic).

Both urinary retention and urinary incontinence are more common as men and women get older. Infections, alcohol, overhydration, dehydration, and certain depression, cold, allergy, opioid medications and general anesthesia medications that cause bladder muscles to relax or the urethra to tighten may lead to temporary cases of urinary retention or incontinence. Surgery, radiation therapy, and a tumor anywhere along the urinary tract that can obstruct the normal flow of urine may also cause persistent urinary retention or incontinence.

How are Urinary Retention and Urinary Incontinence Treated by Conventional Medicine?

Urinary retention treatment interventions include catheter placement to drain urine from the bladder and medications such as hormone therapy, antibiotics for the prevention of urinary tract infection, 5-alpha-reductase inhibitors, or alpha blockers. In more severe cases of urinary retention, surgery either to remove a blockage so urine can flow normally from the bladder or surgery for the placement of a shunt or stent to widen the urinary tract may be recommended.

Urinary incontinence can generally be treated with fluid management, bladder training, pelvic floor exercises, electrical stimulation, and medications, such as anticholinergics, topical estrogen, and tricyclic antidepressants. If other treatments are not working, surgery may be recommended. Protective devices, such as bed pads, diapers, and underwear liners for urinary incontinence management may be suggested.

Integrative Approaches to Urinary Retention and Urinary Incontinence

The integrative approach to urinary retention and incontinence often relies on touch therapies and yoga alongside conventional recommendations. For urinary retention, begin with the massage techniques over the course of the day. For urinary incontinence, begin with either acupressure and/or reflexology. Consider visiting a licensed massage therapist or acupuncturist for more chronic conditions or prevention. Yoga pelvic floor exercises may provide additional benefit for relief of both urinary incontinence and retention.

Before adding any integrative therapy to your treatment plan, speak with your doctor about the benefits and risks. A summary of risks may be found in the Introduction along with detailed instructions for the application of and considerations for each of the indicated therapies.

Integrative Medicine in Action

Patient Story
Integrative Medicine Plan for Urinary Retention:
Acupressure and Yoga.

Patient: Michael, an 81-year old man with bladder cancer experiencing urinary retention.

Chief Complaint: Michael experienced acute periods of urinary retention that could be managed by monitoring his fluid intake. However, following surgery he began to have more persistent urinary retention which was leading to swelling of his ankles.

Treatment: Michael began performing acupressure every time he felt the urge to urinate. He began practicing yoga particularly twisting, standing, and sitting postures to help completely empty his bladder. Michael found yoga was particularly helpful when he did not feel his bladder was completely empty after urinating. In these cases, Michael would practice the yoga sequence one to two times before returning to the restroom.

Outcome: Although his urinary retention did not completely subside, he was overall less symptomatic, and he felt in more control of the urinary retention. The integrative approach assisted in preventing catheter placement.

Chinese Medicine/Acupressure

In Chinese medicine, the Bladder serves to hold and eventually discharge urine in order to rid the body of waste. The ability for the Bladder to perform this function relies largely on the health of other organ systems especially the Kidney. If the Kidneys become weak by cancer therapy, the mechanism by which the Bladder stores and discharges urine can become compromised. There are many other imbalances that can occur in the body and result in urinary symptoms. The recommended acupressure points may help to alleviate symptoms of retention or incontinence.

For urinary retention, apply the recommended points below when there is difficulty in starting to urinate or when urination feels incomplete.

Acupressure

Urinary Retention
Most frequently used (Appendix A)
Kid 10, Ren 3, SP 6, ST 28, UB 28
If accompanied by edema, add: Ren 9, SP 9, UB 20, UB 23
If urination is painful, possibly with blood in the urine, add: GB 26, Kid 5, LI 4, SP 10

Urinary Incontinence
You can use the points below for frequent urination, dribbling after completion or incontinence.
Most frequently used (Appendix A)
DU 20, Kid 7, Ren 4, ST 36, UB 23
If urination is frequent, urgent, burning and dark in color, add: HT 5, Liv 5, SP 6
If frequency is worsened with stress and anxiety, add: HT 7
If frequency is worse at night, add: DU 4, Kid 3
If incontinence with coughing, sneezing or exertion, add: LU 7, SP 6

Homeopathy

Homeopathic remedies may be combined with touch therapies. The timing and dose will vary with each remedy. If you are not experiencing any relief within 2 to 4 weeks, discontinue supplementation.

Urinary Retention
• Causticum. Begin with a dose of 6c, 3 times per day until relief is experienced. Then change the dose to 12c, 2 times per day for the same period of time it took to experience initial relief. Continue with a maintenance therapy is 30c, once per day.
• Sepia. 6c, 3 times per day until relief is experienced. Begin with 12c, 2 times per day for the same period of time it took to experience initial relief. Afterwards, continue with a maintenance dose of 30c, once per day.
• **Staphysagria.** Use this remedy for acute conditions. Begin with 200c until relief is experienced.

Urinary Incontinence

• **Conium.** 6c, 3 times per day for 2 to 4 weeks until symptoms begin to resolve. After 4 weeks, begin with 12 c, 3 times per day for another 2 to 4 weeks. Continue with 30c, once per day for a maintenance dose.

Massage

Massage is best indicated for urinary retention and not for urinary incontinence. Massage when you are beginning to feel symptoms of discomfort. Massage as needed throughout the day. Information on the recommended massage techniques may be found in Chapter 4.

Massage by a Caregiver

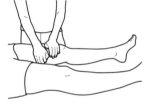 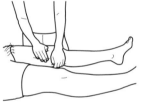 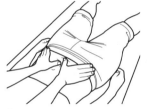

1 Have the person lie on their back, begin by massaging the inner thigh muscles (the adductor magnus and longus) using a twisting style petrissage motion.

2 Use this technique from upper inner thigh to the inner knee.

3 Using circular petrissage motions, massage the lower belly below the belly button in between the hip bones.

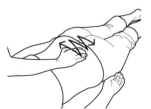 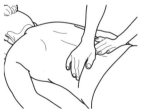

4 Have the person turn over and lie on their belly. Massage the sacrum (triangle shaped bone on the bottom of the spine) area with "brushing" technique.

5 Gently nish with small petrissage strokes on the lower back.

6 Repeat as needed.

Self Massage

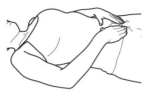 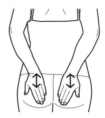

1 Massage the lower belly with both hands using small circular petrissage motions. This is the area below the belly button in between the hip bones. You can do this by putting one hand over the other and massage with one hand. The direction of the circular motion is either direction that is most comfortable. Repeat this technique for one to two minutes.

2 With both hands, palms facing down, reach around to your sacrum (triangle shaped bone on the bottom of the spine) and with a brushing technique, move your hands up and down over the sacrum. Repeat this technique for one to two minutes.

3 Repeat as needed.

Reflexology

For both urinary retention and incontinence, apply reflexology to bring equilibrium to the bladder. Reflexology can be applied throughout the day, as needed. The bladder points can be accessed alone or in conjunction with the other points. Information on reflexology technique can be found in Chapter 4.

Urinary Retention & Urinary Incontinence

Foot Points
H: Pituitary reflexes
R: Adrenal, bladder, kidney reflexes
T: Lumbar, ureter tube reflexes

Hand Points
H: Pituitary reflexes
R: Bladder, kidney reflexes
T: Spinal, ureter tube reflexes

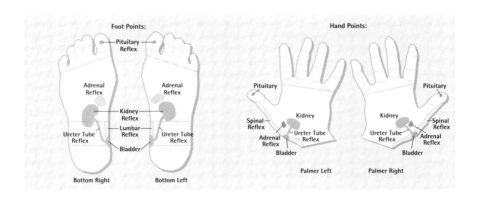

Yoga

The suggested yoga poses physically allow you to work on the muscles around the urethra or urinary canal. For urinary incontinence, the yoga poses put you in an ideal position to strengthen these muscles. For urinary retention, the yoga poses squeeze and open the urinary canal. Use these yoga poses throughout the day as needed.

Breathing (Appendix D): Kapalabhati

Urinary Retention

Poses (Appendix D): Standing forward bend, cobbler's pose, straight leg seated spinal twist, camel pose, supine twist, shoulderstand, supine knee squeeze, relaxation pose

Urinary Incontinence

While holding the postures listed below, squeeze the muscles around the urinary canal

Poses (Appendix D): Mountain pose, chair pose, cobbler's pose, seated forward bend, relaxation pose

Appendices

Appendix A

Acupressure Point Instruction and Illustrations

(Illustrations reprinted from *A Manual of Acupuncture* by kind permission of the Journal of Chinese Publications: www.jcm.co.uk)

Cun Measurements

A common way to locate acupuncture points is through a unit of measurement called cun. Our entire body is proportionate to itself, so that a cun measurement is different for each of us. Use these measurements to help locate the acupoints.

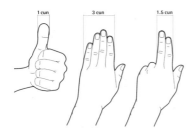

1 cun = the width of the knuckle of the thumb
1.5 cun = the width of the knuckles of the index and middle fingers
3 cun = the width of the knuckles of all four fingers

Illustrated Acupoints

DU Points

DU 4

Lie face down or sit up straight in a chair. Place hands on the top of the hips (just below the waist). The thumbs should be in a straight line across the back (perpendicular to the spine). Try to have the thumbs touch at the spine. From where the thumbs meet, move up one bone. The point is located on the spine, directly below that bone.

Chapters: Constipation, Diarrhea, Pain, Urinary Retention & Incontinence

DU 14

Begin at the protruding bone at the base of the neck. DU 14 is the second big bone you feel working downward just below the base of the neck.

Tip: It can be difficult to locate specific bones of the spine. If you are unsure if you are in the correct location, apply light acupressure to the points below each of the bones on the lower neck.

Chapter: Mouth Sores

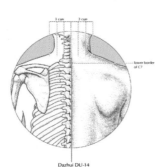

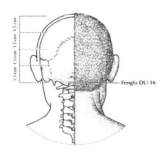

DU 16

Identify the midline of the back of the neck at the hairline. DU 16 is directly above the hairline. You will feel a "dip" above the hairline before touching the skull bone.

Tip: If you have no hairline, begin at the first bone of the spine. Move upwards toward your head in a straight line. DU 16, is the first "dip" you feel.

Chapter: Fatigue

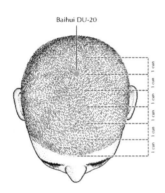

DU 20

This point is located on the midline on the top of the head. Imagine a line connecting the top of each ear. DU 20 is slightly behind the midpoint of this line on the top of the head.

Chapters: Chemo Brain, Depression, Fatigue, Headache, Urinary Retention & Incontinence

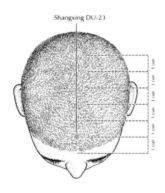

DU 23

Identify the midline of the head. DU 23 is about one thumb's width back from the front hairline.

Tip: If the person has no hairline, simply go one thumb's width from the top of the forehead. To find the top of the forehead, have the person lift their eyebrows. The hairline begins approximately where the wrinkles on the forehead end.

Chapter: Headache

GB Points

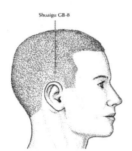

GB 8

GB8 is on the either side of head, one thumb's width above the top of the ear.

Chapter: Headache

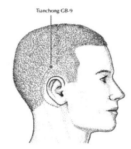

GB 9

GB 9 is located on either side of the head, one thumb's width above the top of the ear and half a thumb's width back.

Chapter: Anxiety & Stress

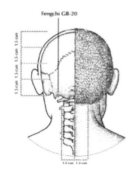

GB 20

Identify the midline of the head. GB 20 is located on the back of the head, just below the skull, about three finger widths to the right or left from the midline.

Tip: It is recommended to apply pressure to the entire area since it is difficult to find the exact location.

Chapters: Fatigue, Headache, Hot Flashes, Pain,

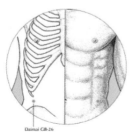

GB 26

GB 26 is located on the lower abdomen, directly above the highpoint of the hip bone, and level with the belly button.

Tip: This point is located directly below Liv 13.

Chapter: Urinary Retention & Incontinence

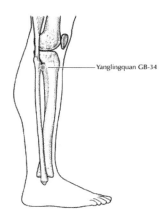

GB 34

Begin below the round bone of the outer knee. GB 34 is located on the outside of the lower leg just below the knee bone.

Tip: It is easiest to locate this point with the knee bent.

Chapters: Constipation, Diarrhea, Fatigue, Headache, Loss of Appetite, Pain, Peripheral Neuropathy

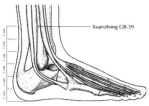

GB 39

Begin at the ankle bone. GB 39 is located on outside lower leg. Move four finger widths upwards along the bone. Now, move one thumb's width toward the back of the leg.

Tip: The exact location of this point lies in the "dip" between the leg bone and the tendons.

Chapter: Headache

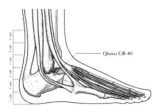

GB 40

Begin at the middle of the ankle bone. GB 40 is located on the outside of the foot, one thumb's width below the ankle bone.

Tip: This point is located on the outside of the tendon just next to the ankle bone.

Chapters: Insomnia, Peripheral Neuropathy

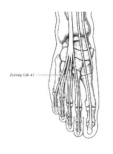

GB 41

Begin on the top of the foot. GB 41 is located approximately two thumb widths above the web between the fourth and fifth toe.

Tip: Follow your finger straight back. The point is on the outside of the tendon of the little toe.

Chapter: Headache

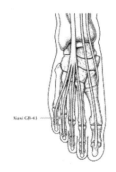

GB 43

Begin on the top of the foot. GB 43 is located at the beginning of the web of the fourth and fifth toe.

Chapter: Headache

HT Points

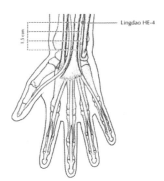

HT 4

Face your palm up. HT 4 is on the inner portion of the forearm, directly above the little finger, about two finger widths above the wrist crease.

Chapter: Anxiety & Stress

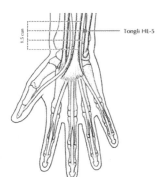

HT 5

Face your palm up. HT 5 is on the inner portion of the forearm, directly above the little finger, about one thumb's width above the wrist crease.

Chapters: Anxiety & Stress, Fatigue, Insomnia, Mouth Sores, Urinary Retention & Incontinence

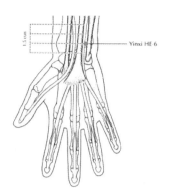

HT 6

Face your palm up. HT 6 is on the inner portion of the forearm, directly above the little finger, about ½ a thumb's width above the wrist crease.

Chapters: Anxiety & Stress, Hot Flashes

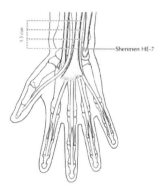

HT 7

Face your palm up. HT 7 is on the inner portion of the forearm, directly above the little finger, on the wrist crease.

Chapters: Anxiety & Stress, Chemo Brain, Depression, Fatigue, Insomnia, Loss of Libido, Shortness of Breath, Urinary Retention & Incontinence

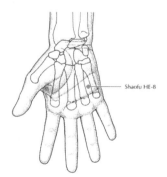

HT 8

Face your palm up. HT 8 is at the spot where the little finger rests when a loose fist is made.

Chapters: Anxiety & Stress, Dry Mouth, Hot Flashes, Insomnia, Mouth Sores

Kid Points

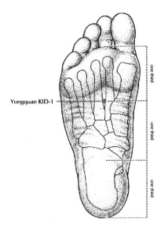

Kid 1

Begin on the sole of the foot. Kid 1 is found in line with the second toe in the dip below the ball of the foot.

Chapters: Anxiety & Stress, Headache, Hot Flashes

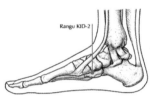

Kid 2

Begin at the front of the inner ankle bone. Slide your finger straight down (towards the toes) to just below the foot bone. As you slide forward, Kid 2 is located on the first dip below the foot bone.

Chapter: Mouth Sores

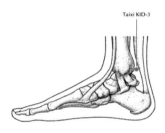

Kid 3

Begin at the ankle bone. Slide your finger backwards (towards the Achilles tendon), Kid 3 is located midway between the tip of the inner ankle bone and the Achilles tendon.

Chapters: Chemo Brain, Depression, Diarrhea, Fatigue, Hot Flashes, Immune Suppression, Insomnia, Loss of Appetite, Shortness of Breath, Urinary Retention & Incontinence

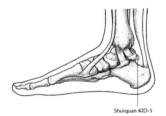

Kid 5

Begin at the ankle bone. Slide your finger backwards (towards the Achilles tendon). Kid 5 is located one thumb's width down from the midpoint of the inner ankle bone and the Achilles tendon.

Chapter: Urinary Retention & Incontinence

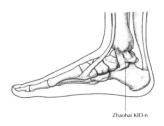

Zhaohai KID-6

Kid 6

Begin at the ankle bone. Kid 6 is located directly below the lowest tip of the inner ankle bone.

Chapters: Depression, Hot Flashes, Loss of Appetite, Shortness of Breath

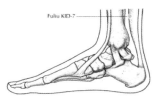

Fuliu KID-7

Kid 7

Begin at the ankle bone. Slide your fingers towards the back of the leg, midway between the inner ankle bone and Achilles tendon. Kid 7 is located two thumb widths above this point.

Chapters: Chemo Brain, Depression, Fatigue, Hot Flashes, Loss of Libido, Pain, Urinary Retention & Incontinence

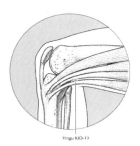

Yingu KID-10

Kid 10

Begin with your knees bent. Kid 10 is located on the inside of the back of the knee, between the two tendons.

Chapter: Urinary Retention & Incontinence

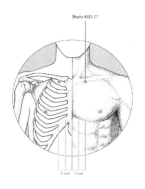

Shufu KID-27

Kid 27

Kid 27 is located on the chest, directly below the collar bone, two thumb widths from the midline.

Chapters: Anxiety & Stress, Shortness of Breath

LI Points

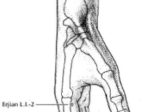

LI 2

LI 2 is located on the thumb side of the index finger. The point is in the depression above the knuckle.

Tip: Locate this point with the finger slightly flexed.

Chapter: Mouth Sores

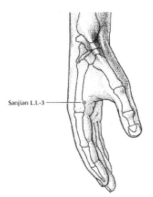

LI 3

LI 3 is located on the thumb side of the index finger, in the depression immediately below the knuckle.

Tip: Locate when a loose fist is made.

Chapter: Dry Mouth

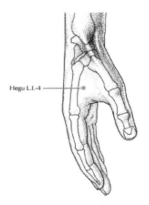

LI 4

LI 4 is located on the bone directly above the middle of the web between the thumb and index finger.

Chapters: Anxiety & Stress, Constipation, Depression, Diarrhea, Dry Mouth, Headache, Hot Flashes, Mouth Sores, Pain, Peripheral Neuropathy, Urinary Retention & Incontinence

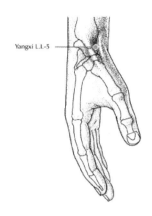

LI 5

Open your hand with the palm facing the floor, fingers spread apart. LI 5 is located in the depression slightly above the inside wrist bone in between the two tendons of the thumb.

Chapter: Peripheral Neuropathy

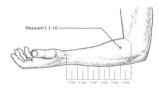

LI 10

Bend your arm in a 90 degree angle. Begin at the outer elbow crease. LI 10 is located two finger widths down from the outer elbow crease.

Chapters: Fatigue, Peripheral Neuropathy

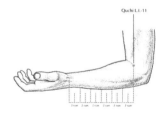

LI 11

Bend your arm in a 90 degree angle. Begin at the elbow crease. LI 11 is located at the end of the outer elbow crease. It is before feeling the elbow bone.

Chapters: Constipation, Diarrhea, Dry Mouth, Hot Flashes

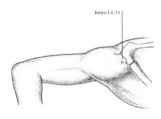

LI 15

Locate this point with the arm raised as depicted in the picture. Begin at the top of the shoulder. LI 15 is located in the depression located slightly in front of and below the shoulder bone.

Chapters: Fatigue, Peripheral Neuropathy

Liv Points

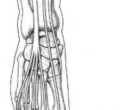

Liv 1

Liv 1 is located on the big toe, directly below the inside corner of the nail.

Chapter: Anxiety & Stress

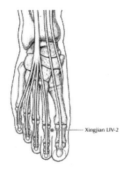

Liv 2

Liv 2 is located on the inside of the big toe at the beginning of the web between the 1st and 2nd toes.

Chapters: Depression, Hot Flashes, Insomnia, Loss of Appetite

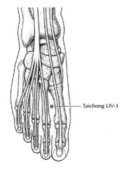

Liv 3

Liv 3 is located on the top of the foot, approximately one thumb's width above the web of the first and second toes.

Chapters: *Anxiety & Stress, Depression, Diarrhea, Fatigue, Headache, Hot Flashes, Insomnia, Loss of Appetite, Peripheral Neuropathy*

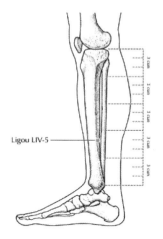

Ligou LIV-5

Liv 5

Liv 5 is located on the inside of the lower leg, five thumb widths above the ankle, on the inside edge behind the leg bone.

Chapters: Loss of Libido, Urinary Retention & Incontinence

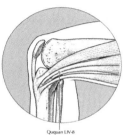

Ququan LIV-8

Liv 8

Begin with the knee bent. Liv 8 is located on the inner side of the knee, directly above the tendons felt at the bottom of the knee, directly behind the knee bone.

Chapters: Fatigue, Hot Flashes, Loss of Libido

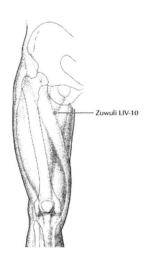

Zuwuli LIV-10

Liv 10

Lie face up. Liv 10 is located four finger widths below the upper border of the pubic bone on the inside of the thigh.

Tip: It is recommended to apply pressure to the entire area since it is difficult to find the exact location.

Chapter: Loss of Libido

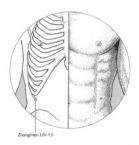

Zhangmen LIV-13

Liv 13

Begin at the bottom of the sternum. Follow the rib cage towards the side of the body. Liv 13 is located directly below the end of the 11th rib.

Chapter: Fatigue

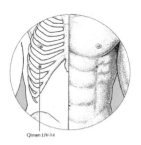

Qimen LIV-14

Liv 14

Liv 14 is located four finger widths out from the bottom of the sternum, directly below the nipple in the sixth rib space.

Caution: Only use light acupressure on the ribcage.

Chapter: Fatigue

LU Points

Zhongfu LU-1

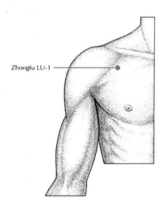

LU 1

Begin at the end of the collar bone. LU 1 is the tender point located in the dip about one thumb's width under the end of the collar bone.

Caution: Only light pressure should be applied on the ribcage.

Chapters: Depression, Dry Mouth, Shortness of Breath

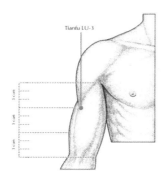

LU 3

LU 3 is between the shoulder and elbow crease. This point is on the outside of the upper portion of the biceps muscle about one third of the way down to the elbow.

Chapter: Depression

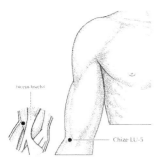

LU 5

Bend your elbow. LU 5 is located on the elbow crease, on the outer side of the tendon.

Chapter: Dry Mouth

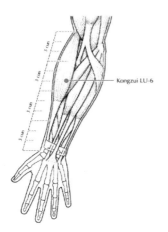

LU 6

Bend your elbow with palm up. LU 6 is located five thumb widths down from the outer elbow crease.

Chapters: Mouth Sores, Shortness of Breath

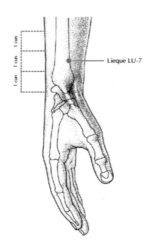

LU 7

Begin in the middle of the thumb knuckle. Pass your finger over the wrist bone and continue up toward the elbow. LU 7 is about one finger's width up from the wrist bone.

Chapters: Fatigue, Hot Flashes, Shortness of Breath, Urinary Retention & Incontinence

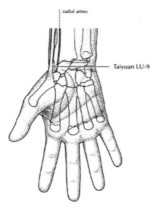

LU 9

LU 9 is located directly below the base of the thumb. Move towards the bottom wrist crease where a pulse is felt.

Chapters: Fatigue, Shortness of Breath

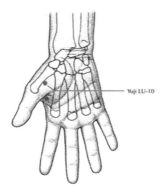

LU 10

This point is located in between the bone and the fleshy part of the thumb skin. LU 10 is at the midpoint of the bone.

Chapters: Hot Flashes, Mouth Sores

PC Points

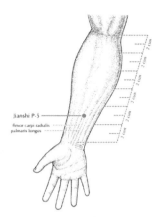

PC 5

Begin on the inside of the forearm with your palm facing up. PC5 is three thumb widths above the wrist crease, on the midline between the two prominent tendons.

Tip: It is easier to locate this point when the hand is in a loose fist.

Chapters: Anxiety & Stress, Dry Mouth, Insomnia Shortness of Breath

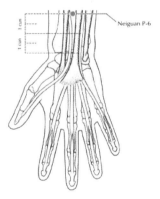

PC 6

Begin on the inside of the forearm with your palm facing up. PC6 is two thumb widths above the wrist crease, on the midline between the two prominent tendons.

Tip: It is easier to locate this point when the hand is in a loose fist.

Chapters: Anxiety & Stress, Diarrhea, Dry Mouth, Fatigue, Headache, Insomnia, Nausea & Vomiting, Shortness of Breath

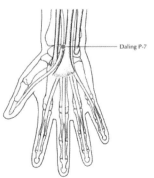

PC 7

Begin on the inside of the forearm with your palm facing up. PC7 is on the midline of wrist crease, between the two prominent tendons.

Tip: It is easier to locate this point when the hand is in a loose fist.

Chapters: Anxiety & Stress, Fatigue, Hot Flashes, Insomnia, Shortness of Breath

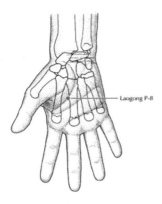

Laogong P-8

PC 8

Face your palm up. Make a loose fist. PC 8 is located in the depression where the middle finger rests on the inside of the palm.

Chapter: Anxiety & Stress

Ren Points

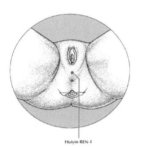

Huiyin REN-1

Ren 1

This point is located between the legs, at the midpoint of the anus and scrotum in men and the anus and rear border of the vagina in women.

Chapter: Loss of Libido

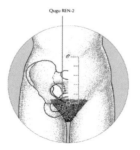

Qugu REN-2

Ren 2

Imagine a line that begins in the middle of the chest and ends at the top of the pubic bone. This line separates the right and left side of the chest and belly. Ren 2 is located on the midline of the belly, directly above the pubic bone.

Chapter: Loss of Libido

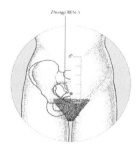

Ren 3

Imagine a line that begins in the middle of the chest and ends at the top of the pubic bone. This line separates the right and left side of the chest and belly. Ren 3 is located on the midline of the belly, one thumb's width above the pubic bone.

Chapter: Urinary Retention & Incontinence

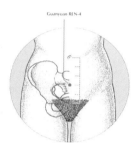

Ren 4

Imagine a line that begins in the middle of the chest and ends at the top of the pubic bone. This line separates the right and left side of the chest and belly. Ren 4 is located four finger widths below belly button.

Chapters: Constipation, Diarrhea, Fatigue, Hot Flashes, Immune Suppression, Pain, Urinary Retention & Incontinence

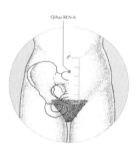

Ren 6

Imagine a line that begins in the middle of the chest and ends at the top of the pubic bone. This line separates the right and left side of the chest and belly. Ren 6 is located on the midline of the abdomen, 1 ½ thumb widths below the belly button.

Chapters: Constipation, Fatigue

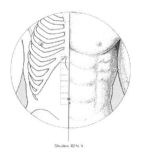

Ren 9

Imagine a line that begins in the middle of the chest and ends at the top of the pubic bone. This line separates the right and left side of the chest and belly. Ren 9 is located on the midline of the belly, one thumb's width above belly button.

Chapters: Dry Mouth, Urinary Retention & Incontinence

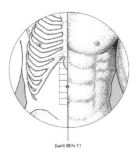

Jianli REN-11

Ren 11

Imagine a line that begins in the middle of the chest and ends at the top of the pubic bone. This line separates the right and left side of the chest and belly. Ren 11 is located on the midline of the belly, three thumb widths above the belly button.

Chapters: Fatigue, Loss of Appetite

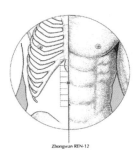

Zhongwan REN-12

Ren 12

Imagine a line that begins in the middle of the chest and ends at the top of the pubic bone. This line separates the right and left side of the chest and belly. Ren 12 is located on the midline of the belly, four thumb widths above the belly button.

Chapters: Anxiety & Stress, Constipation, Dry Mouth, Fatigue, Headache, Insomnia, Loss of Appetite Nausea & Vomiting

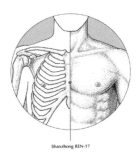

Shanzhong REN-17

Ren 17

Ren 17 is located on the midline of the sternum of the chest on nipple line in men or on the sternum between the breasts in women.

Tip: Apply light pressure above and below the area to find the point that is most tender.

Caution: Only light pressure should be applied on the ribcage.

Chapters: Anxiety & Stress, Depression, Diarrhea, Dry Mouth, Fatigue, Shortness of Breath

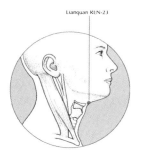

Lianquan REN-23

Ren 23

Ren 23 is located on the neck just above the Adam's apple.

Tip: To find the Adam's apple, place your hand over the area and have the person swallow. You should be able to feel it move up and down.

Caution: Only light acupressure should be applied to the neck and throat area.

Chapter: Dry Mouth

SI Points

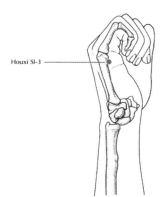

Houxi SI-3

SI 3

SI 3 is located on the side of the hand, below the knuckle of the small finger.

Tip: Locate with a loose fist. The point is not on the palm or the back of the hand.

Chapters: Fatigue, Headache

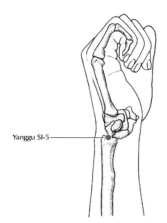

Yanggu SI-5

SI 5

SI 5 is located on the side of the wrist crease, in the dip between the two bones.

Chapter: Peripheral Neuropathy

SJ Points

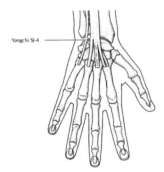

SJ 4

SJ 4 is located just below the wrist crease at the level between the ring and small fingers in the dip.

Chapters: Chemo Brain, Peripheral Neuropathy

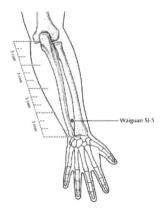

SJ 5

Begin on the top of the forearm. SJ 5 is located two thumb widths above the wrist crease, in the center of the forearm.

Tip: This point is located between the two bones of the arm.

Chapter: Headache

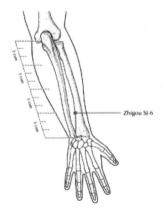

SJ 6

Begin on the top of the forearm. SJ 6 is located three thumb widths above the outer wrist crease, slightly towards the thumb side of the center of the forearm.

Tip: This point is located between the two bones of the arm.

Chapters: Constipation, Fatigue, Pain

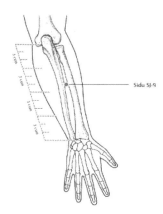

SJ 9

Begin on the top of the forearm. SJ 9 is located seven thumb widths above the outer wrist crease, in the center of the forearm.

Chapter: Peripheral Neuropathy

SP Points

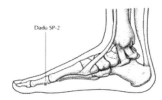

SP 2

SP 2 is located on the side of the foot, in front of the big toe joint.

Chapter: Mouth Sores

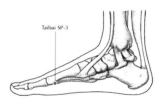

SP 3

SP 3 is located on the side of the foot, behind the big toe joint.

Chapters: Fatigue, Loss of Appetite

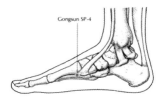

SP 4

SP 4 is located three finger widths behind the big toe joint, towards the ankle on the side of the foot.

Chapters: Hot Flashes, Loss of Appetite, Nausea & Vomiting

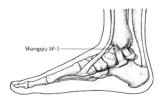

SP 5

SP 5 is located in the dip just in front of the inside ankle bone.

Chapter: Peripheral Neuropathy

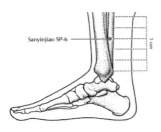

SP 6

SP 6 is located on the inside of the lower leg, in the depression four finger widths above the tip of the ankle, behind the shin bone.

Chapters: Anxiety & Stress, Constipation, Diarrhea, Headache, Hot Flashes, Immune Suppression, Insomnia, Loss of Appetite, Pain, Urinary Retention & Incontinence

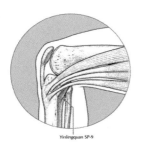

SP 9

Begin on the inside of the shin bone just above the ankle. Slide your finger along the inside of the bone towards the knee cap. SP 9 is located in the dip below the inside of the knee, just behind the shin bone.

Tip: It is recommended to apply pressure to the entire area since it is difficult to find the exact location.

Chapters: Diarrhea, Loss of Appetite, Pain, Shortness of Breath, Urinary Retention & Incontinence

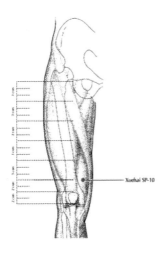

SP 10

Begin on the inside top of the knee cap. SP 10 is located two thumb widths above the inner corner of the kneecap.

Tip: With the knee bent, cup the right palm over the left kneecap. Keep your fingers in a relaxed position (do not spread the fingers unnaturally). The point is located approximately under where the thumbnail falls. It is recommended to apply pressure to the entire area since it is difficult to find the exact location.

Chapters: Headache, Pain, Urinary Retention & Incontinence

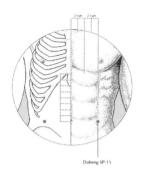

Daheng SP-15

SP 15

SP 15 is located four thumb widths out from the belly button.

Chapter: Diarrhea

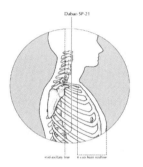

Dabao SP-21

SP 21

SP 21 is located on the side of the chest, halfway between the armpit and the bottom of the rib cage.

Tip: The point is often found at the bottom of the bra-line in women.

Caution: Only light pressure should be applied on the ribcage.

Chapter: Pain

ST Points

ST 6

ST 6 is located on the bulge that appears when the teeth are clenched. The point is about one finger's width above and in front of the angle of the jaw. Unclench jaw to apply acupressure.

Chapter: Dry Mouth

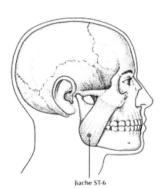

Jiache ST-6

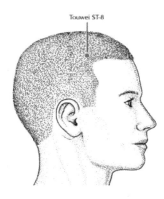

ST 8

Identify the midline of the head. ST 8 is located 4 ½ finger widths from the midline of the head just above the hairline.

Tip: If the person has no hairline, simply go ½ finger's width from the top of the forehead.

Chapter: Headache

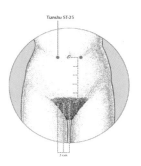

ST 25

ST 25 is located on the belly, two thumb widths out from the belly button.

Chapters: Constipation, Diarrhea, Fatigue

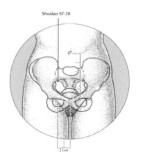

ST 28

ST 28 is located on the belly, two thumb widths out from the belly button and three thumb widths down.

Chapter: Urinary Retention & Incontinence

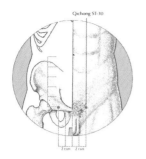

ST 30

Begin at the pubic bone. Imagine a line that begins in the middle of the chest and ends at the top of the pubic bone. ST 30 is on the lower belly, directly above the upper border of the pubic bone, three finger widths out from the midline.

Chapter: Loss of Libido

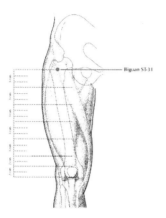

ST 31

Locate this point in a sitting position. Place your finger on the hip bone. Cross one leg sitting Indian style. Slide the finger below and towards the outside of the hip bone. ST 31 is located in the dip behind the muscle that bulges in this position.

Chapters: Fatigue, Peripheral Neuropathy

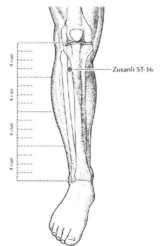

ST 36

ST 36 is located on the outside of the front of the lower leg, four finger widths below the bottom of the kneecap and a finger's width towards the outside of the leg out from the crest of the bone.

Chapters: Chemo Brain, Constipation, Depression, Fatigue, Headache, Immune Suppression, Insomnia, Loss of Appetite, Nausea & Vomiting, Shortness of Breath, Urinary Retention & Incontinence

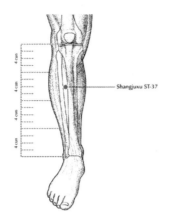

ST 37

ST 37 is located on the outside of the front of the lower leg, eight finger widths below the bottom of the kneecap and a finger's width towards the outside of the leg out from the crest of the bone.

Chapters: Constipation, Diarrhea

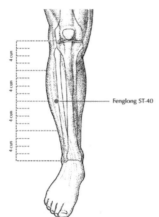

ST 40

ST 40 is located on the outer side of the lower leg, halfway between the outer ankle bone and bottom of the kneecap. The point is two finger widths from the bone.

Chapters: Chemo Brain, Dry Mouth, Headache, Nausea & Vomiting, Pain, Shortness of Breath

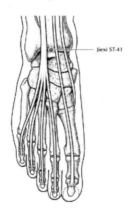

ST 41

Imagine a line connecting the tops of the inner and outer ankle bones. ST 41 is located in the middle of the line in the dip between tendons.

Chapters: Fatigue, Peripheral Neuropathy

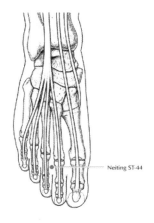

Neiting ST-44

ST 44

ST 44 is located on the foot beginning of the web between the 2nd and 3rd toes.

Chapters: Constipation, Dry Mouth, Headache, Mouth Sores, Nausea/Vomiting

UB Points

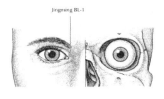

Jingming BL-1

UB 1

UB1 is located just above the inner corner of the eye. Eyes should be closed when applying acupressure to this point.

Caution: Only use light pressure at UB 1.

Chapter: Chemo Brain

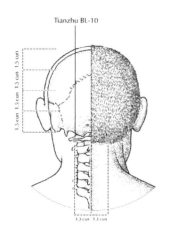

Tianzhu BL-10

UB 10

UB 10 is located on the back of the head, just below the skull, two finger's width from the midline.

Tip: It is recommended to apply pressure to the entire area since it is difficult to find the exact location.

Chapter: Chemo Brain

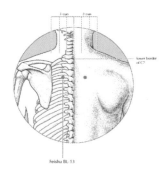

Feishu BL-13

UB 13

Locate the protruding bone at the base of the neck. Count down three bones along the spine. UB 13 is located in the muscle, two finger widths out from the spine.

Tip: It is easier to count the back bones with the head bent slightly forward. The point is approximately level with the top of the shoulder blade. It is recommended to apply pressure to the entire area since it is difficult to find the exact location.

Chapters: Depression, Shortness of Breath

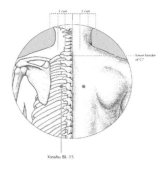

Xinshu BL-15

UB 15

Locate the protruding bone at the base of the neck. Count down five bones along the spine. UB 15 is located in the muscle, two finger widths out from the spine.

Tip: It is easier to count the back bones with the head bent slightly forward. The point is approximately level with the middle of the shoulder blade. It is recommended to apply pressure to the entire area since it is difficult to find the exact location.

Chapters: Anxiety & Stress, Hot Flashes, Insomnia

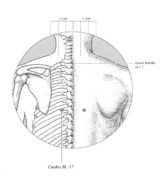

Geshu BL-17

UB 17

Locate the protruding bone at the base of the neck. Count down seven bones along the spine. UB 17 is located in the muscle, two finger widths out from the spine.

Tip: It is easier to count the back bones with the head bent slightly forward. The point is approximately level with the lower end of the shoulder blade. It is recommended to apply pressure to the entire area since it is difficult to find the exact location.

Chapter: Fatigue

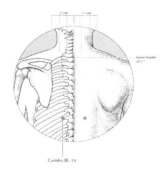

Ganshu BL-18

UB 18

Locate the protruding bone at the base of the neck. Count down nine bones along the spine. UB 18 is located in the muscle, two finger widths out from the spine.

Tip: It is easier to count the back bones with the head bent slightly forward. Follow the lower end of the shoulder blade to the spine. Count down two more bones. It is recommended to apply pressure to the entire area since it is difficult to find the exact location.

Chapter: Fatigue

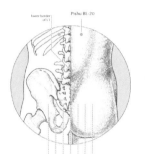

UB 20

Lie face down or sit up straight in a chair. Place hands on the top of the hips (just below the waist). The thumbs should be in a straight line across the back (perpendicular to the spine). Try to have the thumbs touch at the spine. Count up four bones along the spine. UB 20 is located two finger widths out from the spine.

Tip: It is recommended to apply acupressure to the entire area since it is difficult to find the exact location.

Chapters: Fatigue, Urinary Retention & Incontinence

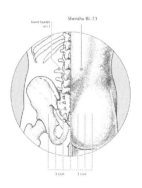

UB 23

Lie face down or sit up straight in a chair. Place hands on the top of the hips (just below the waist). The thumbs should be in a straight line across the back (perpendicular to the spine). Try to have the thumbs touch at the spine. Count up one bone along the spine. UB 23 is located two finger widths out from the spine.

Tip: It is recommended to apply pressure to the entire area since it is difficult to find the exact location.

Chapters: Depression, Diarrhea, Fatigue, Hot Flashes, Pain, Shortness of Breath, Urinary Retention & Incontinence

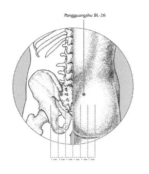

UB 28

Lie face down or sit up straight in a chair. Place hands on the top of the hips (just below the waist). The thumbs should be in a straight line across the back (perpendicular to the spine). Try to have the thumbs touch at the spine. Count down three thumb widths along the spine and onto the tailbone. UB 28 is located in the "dip" two finger widths out from the tailbone.

Chapter: Urinary Retention & Incontinence

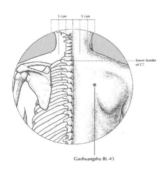

UB 43

Locate the protruding bone at the base of the neck. Count down four bones along the spine. UB 43 is located on the edge of the shoulder blade, four finger widths out from the spine.

Tip: It is easier to count the back bones with the head bent slightly forward. It is recommended to apply pressure to the entire area since it is difficult to find the exact location.

Chapter: Immune Suppression

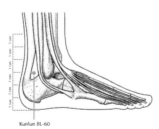

UB 60

Begin at the ankle bone. Slide your finger backwards (towards the Achilles tendon), UB 60 is located midway between the tip of the outer ankle bone and the Achilles tendon.

Chapter: Headache

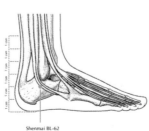

UB 62

Begin at the ankle bone. UB 62 is located approximately 1/2 a thumb's width directly below the outer ankle bone.

Chapter: Fatigue

Additional Points

An Mian

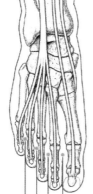

Begin at the bone directly behind the ear on either side of the head. An Mian is located in the "dip" at the bottom part of this bone.

Tip: It is recommended to apply pressure to the entire area since it is difficult to find the exact location.

Chapter: Insomnia

Anmian (N-HN-54)

Ba Feng

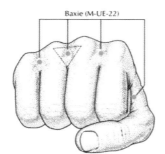

Ba Feng are four points located on the top of each foot, just above the web of the toes.

Tip: These points overlap in location with ST 44, Liv 2 & GB 43.

Chapter: Peripheral Neuropathy

Bafeng (M-LE-8)

Ba Xie

Baxie (M-UE-22)

Make a fist. Ba Xie are four points located in the "dips" just above the web of the fingers.

Chapter: Peripheral Neuropathy

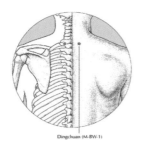

Dingchuan (M-BW-1)

Ding Chuan

Begin at the protruding bone at the base of the neck. Locate DU 14. Ding Chuan is located approximately one thumb's width out from below that bone.

Chapter: Shortness of Breath

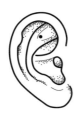

Ear Shenmen

Begin at the top of the ear. Slide finger down and on a diagonal toward the face. Ear Shenmen is located in the triangular depression.

Tip: It is recommended to apply pressure to the entire area since it is difficult to find the exact location.

Chapter: Anxiety & Stress

Sishencong (M-HN-1)

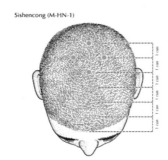

Si Chen Cong

Begin at the top of the head at DU 20. Si Chen Cong are the four points that surround DU 20.

Tip: The four points form a diamond in front of, behind and next to DU 20.

Chapter: Chemo Brain

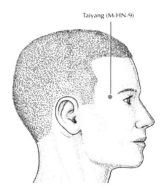

Tai Yang

Begin at the outside of the eye. Tai Yang is located in the "dip" approximately one thumb's width out from the eye, at the temple.

Chapters: Chemo Brain, Headache

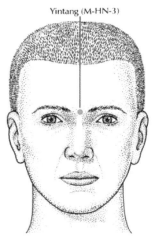

Yin Tang

Yin Tang is located on the forehead, at the midpoint of the inner ends of the eyebrows.

Chapters: Anxiety & Stress, Chemo Brain, Depression, Insomnia

Appendix B
Anatomical Muscle Reference Model

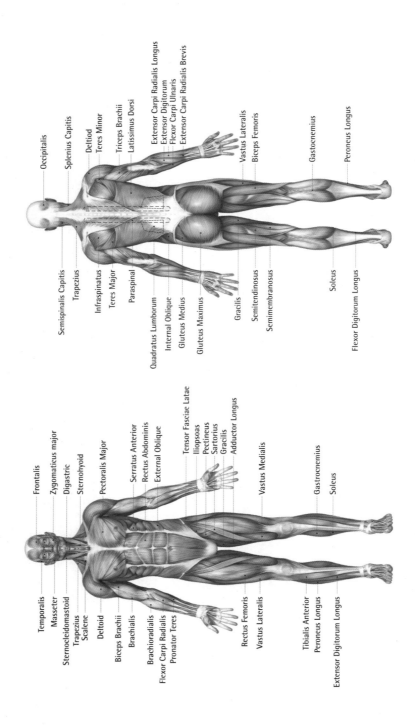

Appendix C
Reflexology Foot and Hand Reference Charts

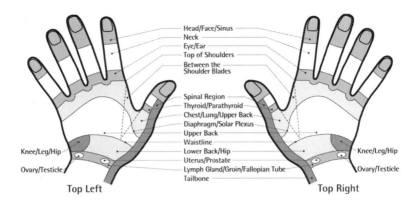

Head/Face/Sinus
Neck
Eye/Ear
Top of Shoulders
Between the
Shoulder Blades

Spinal Region
Thyroid/Parathyroid
Chest/Lung/Upper Back
Diaphragm/Solar Plexus
Upper Back
Waistline
Lower Back/Hip
Uterus/Prostate
Lymph Gland/Groin/Fallopian Tube
Tailbone

Knee/Leg/Hip
Ovary/Testicle

Knee/Leg/Hip
Ovary/Testicle

Top Left   **Top Right**

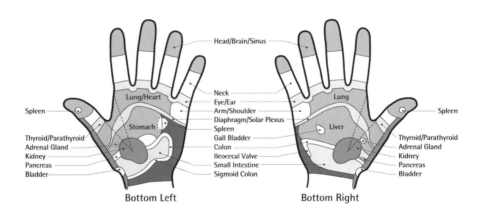

Head/Brain/Sinus

Lung/Heart
Spleen
Stomach

Thyroid/Parathyroid
Adrenal Gland
Kidney
Pancreas
Bladder

Neck
Eye/Ear
Arm/Shoulder
Diaphragm/Solar Plexus
Spleen
Gall Bladder
Colon
Ileocecal Valve
Small Intestine
Sigmoid Colon

Lung
Liver

Spleen

Thyroid/Parathyroid
Adrenal Gland
Kidney
Pancreas
Bladder

Bottom Left   **Bottom Right**

© 2010 Kevin and Barbara Kunz

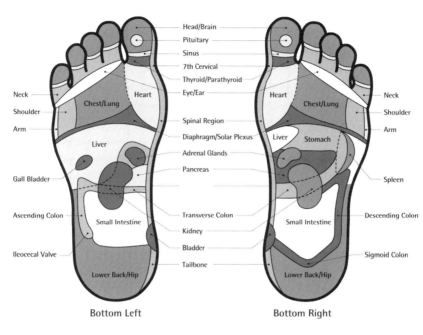

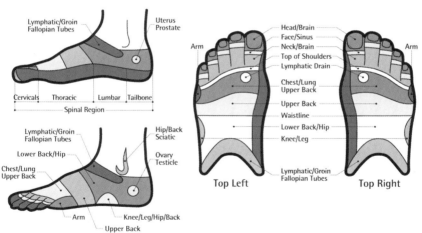

© 2010 Kevin and Barbara Kunz

Appendix D
Yoga Instruction and Illustrations

Contents

Alternate Nostril Breathing
(Anuloma Viloma)

Level: Beginner
Caution: Dizziness, asthma, respiratory problems, and high blood pressure
Recommended: Anxiety & Stress, Chemo Brain, Depression, Diarrhea, Fatigue, Headache, Hot Flashes, Immune Suppression, Insomnia, Loss of Libido, Nausea & Vomiting, Pain, Peripheral Neuropathy

In this breathing exercise, you inhale through one nostril, retain the breath, and then exhale through the other nostril.

1 Come onto the floor and sit in a cross-legged position. Bring your left hand to rest on your left knee and your right hand close to your nostrils. Tucking your right middle and index fingers downwards toward the inside of your palm, place your thumb by your right nostril and your ring and little fingers by your left nostril.

2 Closing your right nostril with your thumb, inhale through your left nostril for a count of four.

3 Closing your left nostril with your ring and little fingers, hold your breath for a count of four.

4 Releasing your thumb from your right nostril, exhale through your right nostril for a count of four, keeping your left nostril closed with your ring and little fingers.

5 Inhale through your right nostril for a count of four.

6 Closing your right nostril with your thumb, hold your breath for a count of four.

7 Releasing your ring and little fingers from your left nostril, exhale through your left nostril for a count of four, keeping your right nostril closed with your thumb. This completes one round of alternate nostril breathing. Repeat, concentrating fully on the breath. Start by practicing three rounds, gradually increasing to 10 rounds of alternate nostril breathing.

Modifications/Props:

• For hip support, sit on a folded blanket. If it is uncomfortable to sit on the floor, come to sit upright on a chair.

• When first learning alternate nostril breathing, do not retain the breath; focus only on the inhalations and exhalations of this breathing exercise.

• As you become more advanced, practice inhaling to four counts, holding for 16 counts, and exhaling for eight counts.

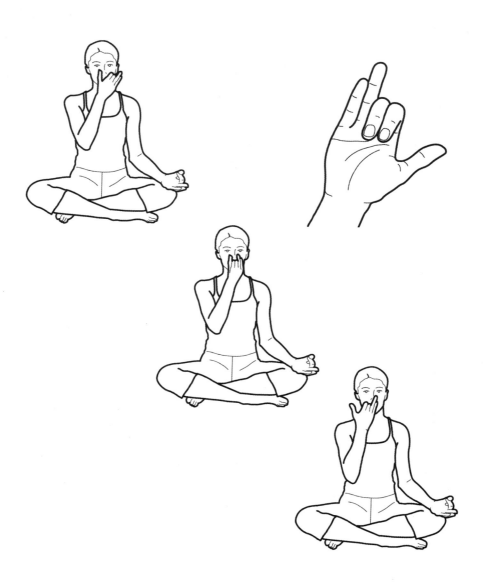

Kapalabhati
(Skull Brightener Breath)

Level: Intermediate
Caution: Dizziness, asthma, respiratory problems, and high blood pressure
Contraindication: Abdominal surgery, hernia, and pregnancy
Recommended: Anxiety & Stress, Constipation, Depression, Fatigue, Immune Suppression, Loss of Appetite, Loss of Libido, Lymphedema, Urinary Retention & Incontinence

Kapalabhati is a highly energizing breathing exercise that consists of exhalations and inhalations followed by breath retention.

1 Come onto the floor and sit in a cross-legged position. Bring both hands to rest on the knees.

2 Inhale fully and exhale completely for two breaths.

3 Inhale to a comfortable level, preparing to begin rhythmic belly contractions.

4 Exhale, pulling the diaphragm up, and begin to force the air out of your lungs with steady and rhythmic contractions (pumping) of the belly muscles. Repeat contractions 15-60 times. Allow the lungs to gently and passively fill with air on the inhalations.

5 Inhale and exhale completely.

6 Inhale fully and hold your breath for as long as you feel comfortable (15 seconds- 1 minute).

7 Slowly exhale completely. Repeat the exercise for three cycles. Gradually build the number of contractions and the length of time you retain your breath. Do not hold your breath; inhalation is natural and should be effortless. If the strength of your exhalation begins to weaken, reduce the number of contractions per cycle.

Modifications/Props:

• For hip support, sit on a folded blanket. If it is uncomfortable to sit on the floor, come to sit upright on a chair.

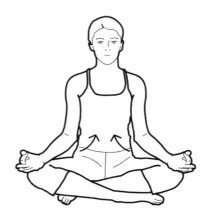

Ujjayi Breath (Conqueror Breath)

Level: Beginner
Caution: Respiratory problems
Recommended: Anxiety & Stress, Chemo Brain, Constipation, Depression,
Fatigue, Headaches, Hot Flashes, Immune Suppression, Insomnia, Loss of Libido,
Loss of Appetite, Lymphedema, Nausea & Vomiting, Peripheral Neuropathy, Pain,
Shortness of Breath

Ujjayi breath is the primary breath technique in yoga. Ujjayi breath can be
practiced on its own or as a deep breathing technique during your yoga posture
practice.

1 Come onto the floor and sit in
a cross-legged position. Bring both
hands to rest on the knees.

2 With lips loosely closed, inhale
slowly through both nostrils, closing
off the glottis (the opening between
the vocal chords). When you achieve
the right breath, you will hear a soft
humming sound. Feel the passage of
the breath expanding the diaphragm
fully. Notice the sensation of your
entire body inflating like a balloon.
Hold for a moment.

3 Exhale gently and completely
through both nostrils until all the
breath is gone. Feel the sensation
of your body deflating. Notice the
stillness. Repeat, concentrating fully
on the breath. Start by practicing five
rounds of Ujjyai breath, gradually
increasing to 20 rounds.

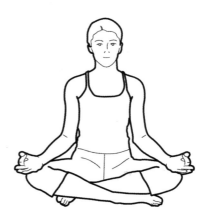

Modifications/Props:

• For hip support, sit on a folded
blanket. If it is uncomfortable to sit
on the floor, come to sit upright on
a chair.

• When first learning Ujjayi breath,
do not hold the breath; focus only
on the inhalations and exhalations of
this breathing exercise.

Sun Salutation (Surya Namaskar)

Level: Intermediate
Caution: Pregnancy (unless experienced with Sun Salutation), and carpal tunnel syndrome
Contraindication: Back injury
Recommended: Chemo Brain, Depression, Fatigue, Immune Suppression, Lymphedema, Pain, Peripheral Neuropathy

Sun Salutation is a sequence of postures (vinyasa) performed as one continuous exercise. A single round of sun salutation consists of two complete sequences: one for the right side of the body and one for the left side of the body. Each posture is coordinated with the breath.

1 Inhale, stand tall in Mountain pose. Exhale, bringing your hands into prayer position. Weight is evenly distributed on both feet.

2 Inhale, raise your arms over your head, bringing fingertips to touch with upper arms alongside your ears. Gently arch back from the waist, as far as it feels comfortable. Neck is relaxed.

3 Exhale, bend forward from your hips, bringing your forehead toward your knees, and press your palms down into the floor. Fingertips are in line with your toes. Bend your knees if needed.

4 Inhale, bring the right leg back into a lunge position, resting your knee and top of the foot on the floor. Arch back slightly and look up, lifting your chin.

5 Exhale, step the left leg back into a high pushup position, supporting your weight with your hands and toes. Keep your head, spine and legs in a straight line. Look at the floor between your hands.

6 Retaining your breath, lower your knees, then chest, and then chin to the floor. Keep your hips up and your toes curled under.

7 Inhale, lower your hips and stretch forward, pointing your toes. Backbend slightly from your waist, using your arms to lift your upper body into Cobra pose. Bend back only as far as it feels comfortable. Look up and back.

8 Exhale, curl your toes under, and raise your hips up to push back into Downward Facing Dog pose (inverted "V" position). Your hands are shoulder-width apart and your feet are hip-width apart. Look at your belly button. Try to bring your heels down to the floor.

9 Inhale, step forward and place your right foot between your hands into a lunge position, resting your left knee and top of the foot on the floor. Arch back slightly and look up, lifting your chin.

10 Exhale, step the left leg forward and bend forward, bringing your forehead toward your knees, pressing your palms down (as in position 3).

11 Inhale, raise your arms over your head, bringing fingertips to touch (as in position 2). Gently arch back from the waist, as far as it feels comfortable. Neck is relaxed.

12 Exhale, gently come back into Mountain pose. Repeat the sequence, stepping with the left leg. Start by practicing three rounds of Sun Salutation, and as you become more advanced, gradually increasing to 10 rounds.

Modifications/Props:

• If at any point you feel tired, come into Child's pose.

• If it is difficult to bring your knee to the floor for lunge position (as in position 4 or position 9), place a folded towel or blanket under your knee when bringing your leg back.

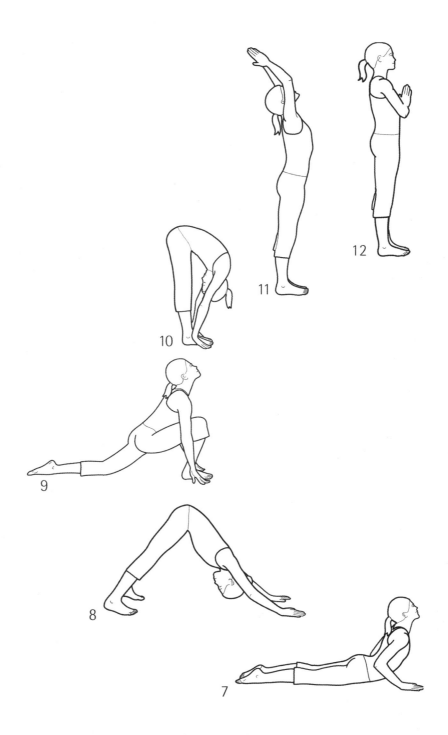

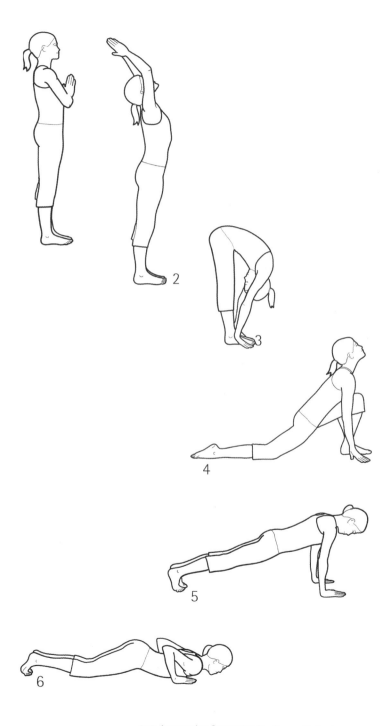

Bow Pose (Dhanurasana)

Level: Advanced
Posture Type: Backbend
Caution: Lower back injury and high or low blood pressure
Contraindication: Neck injury and pregnancy
Recommended: Anxiety & Stress, Constipation, Depression, Fatigue, Immune Suppression, Peripheral Neuropathy

1 Lie on your stomach with your forehead resting on the floor. Bring your arms by your sides behind you with palms facing up. Exhale and bend both knees towards your buttocks. Take hold of the outside of your ankles with your hands. Knees are hip-width apart.

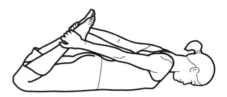

2 Inhale, lift your thighs, head, and chest off the floor. Pull your upper body forward. Back muscles are soft.

3 Exhale, lift your inner thighs up towards the ceiling and press your sacrum down to the floor. Relax your neck and bring your shoulder blades in towards your back. Keep lifting your heels and thighs higher. Look at a point in front of you.

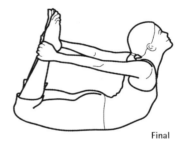

4 Take five deep breaths. Exhale and slowly release, bringing your thighs, chest, ankles, and forehead to the floor. Rest on the floor for a few breaths.

Final

Modifications/Props:

• Fold a blanket under your upper body and upper legs to support lifting your thighs off the floor.

• If you are unable to hold your ankles with your hands, wrap a strap around the top of your ankles. Keeping your arms extended, hold the ends of the strap as you lift your thighs off the floor.

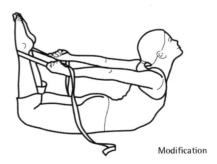

Modification

Bridge Pose
(Setu Bandha Sarvangasana)

Level: Intermediate
Posture Type: Backbend
Caution: Neck injury and high or low blood pressure
Recommended: Anxiety & Stress, Depression, Fatigue, Immune Suppression, Shortness of Breath

1 Come onto the floor. Lie comfortably on your back with your knees bent and feet flat on the floor. Feet are hip-width apart, and knees are directly over your heels. Bring your arms alongside your body with palms facing down.

2 Exhale, lift your hips and buttocks off the floor. Clasp your hands and interlace your fingers and come onto the tops of your shoulders. Your shoulders should be straight and flat to the ground.

3 Take five deep breaths. When you are ready to come out of the pose, exhale and slowly release. Bring your knees to your chest.

Modifications/Props:

• If your shoulders are tense, fold a blanket under your shoulders.

• To make this pose more restorative, place a block or a few pillows under your lower back and come to rest on this support.

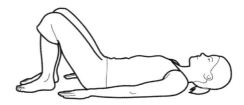

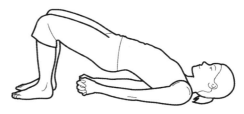

Final

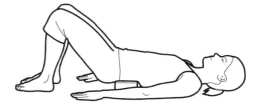

Modification

Camel Pose (Ustrasana)

Level: Advanced
Posture Type: Backbend
Caution: Lower back injury, neck injury, and high or low blood pressure
Recommended: Constipation, Fatigue, Peripheral Neuropathy, Shortness of Breath, Urinary Retention & Incontinence

1 Sit on your heels with your legs hip-distance apart. Come up on your knees and align your hips and thighs so that they are vertical. Press the tops of your feet into the floor. Bring your palms to the tops of your buttocks to support your lower back. Fingertips pointing down.

2 Inhale, push your thighs forward and scoop your sacrum down and under. Relax your buttocks.

3 Exhale, press your shinbones down while lifting your chest up. Allow your head to gently tilt back. Look toward the wall behind you. Be careful not to strain your neck by keeping your neck in a neutral position. To complete the pose, bring your hands to the outside of your heels.

4 Take five deep breaths. Inhale and slowly release by pushing down through your hips. Leading with your chest, gradually lift your head back to a neutral position. Rest in Child's pose for a few breaths.

Modifications/Props:

• If it is difficult to bring your hands to the outside of your heels, keep your palms on the tops of your buttocks.

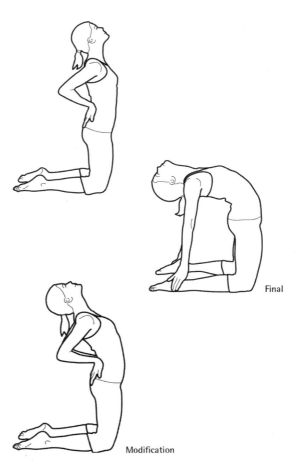

Final

Modification

Chair Pose (Utkatasana)

Level: Beginner
Posture Type: Standing and Balancing
Caution: Knee injury and high or low blood pressure
Recommended: Insomnia, Peripheral Neuropathy, Urinary Retention & Incontinence

1 Stand tall in Mountain pose.

2 Exhale, bend your knees, lowering your body as if you were sitting in a chair, and raise your arms over your head. Arms should be shoulder-width apart and in line with your ears, palms facing each other and fingertips pointing toward the ceiling. Bring your knees together and your thighs parallel to the floor or as close as you can. Lean slightly forward from the waist, so that your knees are directly in line with your toes.

3 Take five deep breaths. When you are ready to come out of the pose, exhale and return to Mountain pose.

Modifications/Props:

• If you need balance support, rest your sacrum on a wall when lowering your body into a sitting position.

• If it is difficult to hold this pose while standing, come into the pose by lowering your body to sit in a chair.

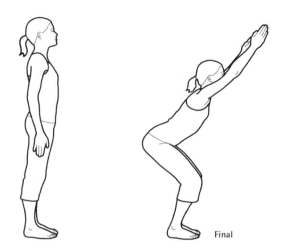

Final

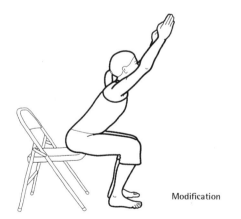

Modification

Child's Pose (Balasana)

Level: Beginner
Posture Type: Seated and Restorative
Caution: Knee injury and pregnancy
Recommended: Anxiety & Stress, Constipation, Nausea & Vomiting, Pain

1 Sit back on your heels, knees hip-width apart.

2 Exhale, bring your upper body between your thighs. Allow your forehead to rest on the floor and bring your arms by your sides with palms facing up.

3 Take 5-10 deep breaths. Inhale and slowly release by lengthening and lifting the upper body back into a neutral kneeling position.

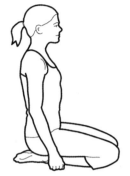

Modifications/Props:

• Fold a blanket between the back of your thighs and calves to support sitting back on your heels.

• If you find it difficult to bend forward, place a pillow or a blanket under your forehead.

• To make the pose more restorative, open your thighs wide and place a folded blanket or pillow under your head, arms, and knees.

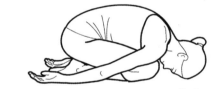

Final

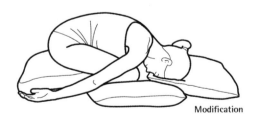

Modification

Cobbler's Pose (Baddha Konasana)

Level: Beginner
Posture Type: Seated
Caution: Pelvic injury and knee injury
Recommended: Loss of Libido, Peripheral Neuropathy, Urinary Retention &
Incontinence

1 Come onto the floor. Sit up tall
with your legs straight in front of you.
Feet are together and hands are flat
on the floor, just behind your hips.
Fingertips are pointing forward.

2 Exhale, bring your feet in as close as
you can towards your pelvis. Dropping
your knees out to the sides, press the
soles of your feet together. Place your
hands on your ankles or feet.

3 Inhale, lengthen your spine.

4 Exhale, fold forward, bringing your
head towards your feet.

5 Take 5-10 deep breaths. When
you are ready to come out of the
pose, slowly sit up, lift your knees, and
extend your legs straight out in front
of you.

Modifications/Props:

• For hip support, sit on a folded
blanket.

• If you are unable to bring your knees
to the floor, place an additional folded
blanket or pillow under each outer
thigh and knee.

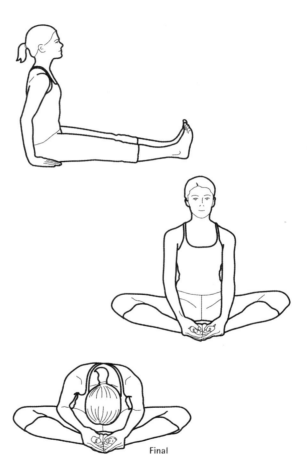

Final

Cobra Pose (Bhujangasana)

Level: Intermediate
Posture Type: Backbend
Caution: Back injury, pregnancy, carpal tunnel syndrome, and high or low blood pressure
Recommended: Anxiety & Stress, Constipation, Depression, Fatigue, Immune Suppression, Peripheral Neuropathy, Shortness of Breath

1 Lie on your stomach with your forehead resting against the floor. Palms are on the floor, and fingertips are in line with your shoulders. Fingers facing forward, elbows bent and tucked into the sides of your body. Legs are stretched back and hip-width apart. Press the tops of the feet and your thighs into the floor.

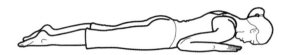

2 Inhale, begin to lift your chest off the floor by drawing your elbows in, straightening your arms, squeezing your thighs and buttocks, and rolling your inner thighs upward. Keep your neck long and in line with your spine. Your shoulders should be away from your ears and shoulder blades should be moving in towards your back. Look up.

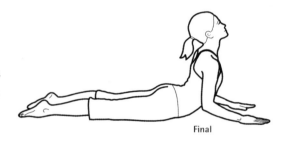

Final

3 Take five deep breaths. Exhale and slowly release to rest on the floor for a few breaths.

Modifications/Props:

• If your body is tense, fold a blanket under your pelvis and lift your chest only two inches off the floor, without straightening your arms. Look toward your nose.

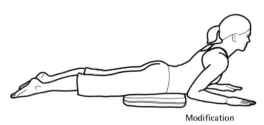

Modification

Dancer's Pose (Natarajasana)

Level: Advanced
Posture Type: Standing, Balancing, and Backbend
Caution: Back injury and high or low blood pressure
Contraindication: Knee injury and ankle injury
Recommended: Peripheral Neuropathy

1 Stand tall in Mountain pose.

2 Inhale, shift your weight onto your right foot. Bend your left leg and bring your left foot backwards towards your left buttock. Grasp your left foot with your left hand around the outside of the foot and bring it as close to your buttock as you can with ease. Contract your right thigh, being careful not to lock your knee, to keep the standing leg straight and strong. Focus your attention on a point in front of you to help keep your balance. Breathe deeply.

3 Slowly, keeping your upper body upright, lift your right arm and lean forward about 45 degrees. Lift the left foot and thigh up behind you, gradually bringing the thigh parallel to the floor.

4 Take three deep breaths. Exhale, slowly release your grasp and place your left foot on the floor. Stand tall in Mountain pose. Repeat on the other side.

Modifications/Props:

• If you need balance support, face a wall and place the hand of your extended arm against it as you bring your foot backwards towards your buttock.

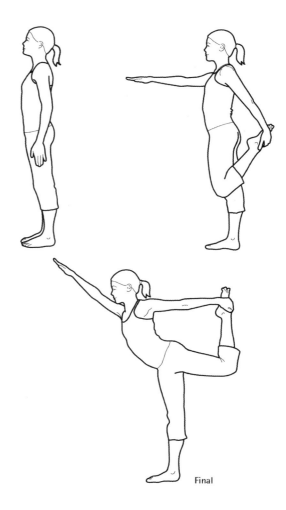

Final

Downward Facing Dog Pose
(Adho Mukha Svanasana)

Level: Beginner
Posture Type: Standing
Caution: Pregnancy, carpal tunnel syndrome, and high or low blood pressure
Recommended: Constipation

1 Come onto the floor on your hands and knees. Palms and fingers spread, hands are in line with your shoulders and are shoulder-width apart. Knees are directly below your hips. Feet hip-width apart, toes are curled under.

2 Exhale, bring your knees off the floor and lift your sacrum up towards the ceiling. Keep your knees slightly bent at first. Shoulders and head are facing down. Look towards your belly button.

3 Inhale and exhale. Gently straighten your legs and try to bring your heels towards the floor. Press your fingertips into the floor and allow your hips to move up and back, coming into an inverted "V" position. Distribute your weight evenly between your hands and feet. Lengthen your back and do not round it. Keep your head between your upper arms.

4 Take 5-10 deep breaths. Exhale, and slowly release to rest in Child's pose.

Modifications/Props:

• If your shoulders are tense, practice the pose in a standing position with the support of a folding chair against a wall. Standing two feet from the seat of the folding chair, hold onto the seat and come into the pose.

• If it is difficult to straighten your legs, keep your knees slightly bent.

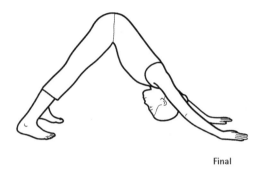

Final

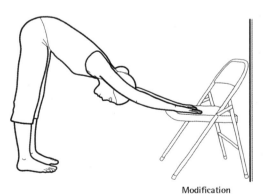

Modification

Fish Pose (Matsyasana)

Level: Intermediate
Posture Type: Backbend
Caution: Lower back injury and high or low blood pressure
Contraindication: Neck injury
Recommended: Shortness of Breath

1 Lie down on your back and come into Relaxation pose. Bring your arms alongside your body with palms facing down. Bringing your elbows in as close as you can under the middle part of your back, tuck your hands beneath your buttocks.

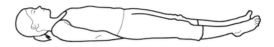

2 Inhale, pressing your forearms and elbows down, lift your upper chest and arch your back. Slowly, allow your head to tilt back. Minimize the amount of weight on your head to avoid crunching your neck.

3 Take five deep breaths. Exhale, bringing your head up and off the ground. Gently lower your chest back down to the floor and rest in Relaxation pose.

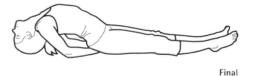

Final

Modifications/Props:

• If your neck or throat is tense in this pose, place a folded blanket under your head for support.

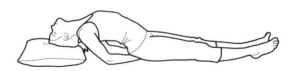

Modification

Headstand (Sirshasana)

Level: Advanced
Posture Type: Inversion
Caution: High or low blood pressure, dizziness, lymphedema, and pregnancy (unless experienced with this pose).
Contraindication: Back injury and neck injury
Recommended: Chemo Brain

1 Come onto the floor. Sit back on your heels and rest in Child's pose.

2 Inhale, sit up on your heels into a kneeling position. Place your forearms on the floor in front of you. Hold your left elbow with your right hand and your right elbow with your left hand.

3 Exhale, rotate your forearms outward and interlock your fingers to form a triangle shape base. Lower the crown of your head so that the top of your head touches the floor. Palms of your hands clasp the back of your head.

4 Inhale, lift your hips above your head and straighten your legs.

5 Exhale, walk your feet toward your head, stretching up high on your toes.

6 Inhale, support your weight through your arms and shoulders as you slowly bend your knees into your chest and lift your feet off the floor.

7 When you feel strong and confident, exhale and straighten your hips by bringing your bent knees to point towards the ceiling.

8 Inhale, push down through your forearms.

9 Exhale, straighten your legs by pressing your heels toward the ceiling. Belly muscles are contracted and toes are slightly pointed.

10 Take 5-10 deep breaths. When you are ready to come out of the pose, exhale, and then bend and lower your knees in towards your chest. Gradually bring your feet to the floor. Sit back on your heels and rest in Child's pose. When first learning this pose, the majority of your weight should be in your shoulders and arms. As you become more comfortable, gradually rest more weight on your head.

Modifications/Props:

• For head and forearm support, place a folded blanket under your forearms.

• If you need balance support, practice this pose against a wall.

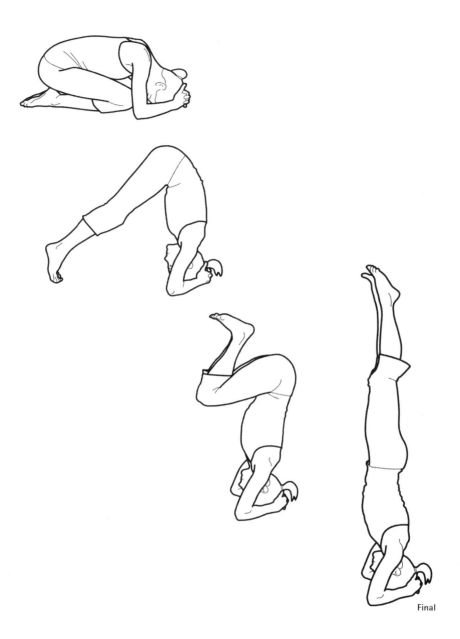

Final

Legs Up Relaxation Pose
(Viparita Karani)

Level: Beginner
Posture Type: Inversion and Restorative
Caution: Neck injury and back injury
Recommended: Headaches, Hot Flashes, Loss of Libido, Lymphedema, Pain

1 Lie near a wall. With legs extended, sit sideways. Exhale, swing your legs up the wall. Rest your legs against the wall so that they form a 45-90 degree angle. Legs muscles are slightly contracted. Relax your arms at your sides, palms up. Release the weight of your thighs and belly. Close your eyes.

2 Take 5-10 deep breaths. When you are ready to come out of the pose, slowly bring your knees toward your belly, roll onto your side, and come into a sitting position.

Modifications/Props:

• This pose requires an upright support or wall.

• If your body is tense, place one or two folded blankets about five inches from the wall. Allow your buttocks to relax into the space between the blankets and wall as your legs rest on the wall.

• If your feet begin to tingle, bend your knees and bring the soles of your feet together. Heels are close to your pelvis.

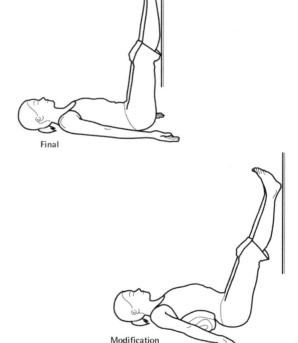

Final

Modification

Mountain Pose (Tadasana)

Level: Beginner
Posture Type: Standing
Caution: None
Recommended: Lymphedema, Peripheral Neuropathy, Shortness of Breath, Urinary Retention & Incontinence

1 Stand as tall as you can without rising onto your toes. Feet are parallel, with your big toes touching. Keep your knees straight, but not locked, and your shoulder blades down. Slightly tilt your pelvis forward to prevent any curvature of the spine at the small of your back. Chin is parallel to the floor. Let your arms hang by your sides with your palms facing towards your body. Weight is evenly distributed.

2 Inhale, bring your hands together in front of your sternum, in prayer position. Exhale, relax your facial muscles. Focus your attention on a point in front of you to keep balanced.

3 Breathe slowly and steadily for 5-10 deep breaths.

Modifications/Props:

• If you want alignment support, stand against a wall with your heels and shoulder blades touching the wall. The back of your head should not touch the wall.

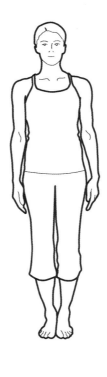

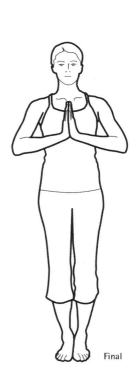

Final

Plough Pose (Halasana)

Level: Advanced
Posture Type: Inversion
Caution: High or low blood pressure, dizziness, lymphedema, and pregnancy (unless experienced with this pose)
Contraindication: Neck injury
Recommended: Anxiety & Stress, Constipation, Depression, Hot Flashes, Immune Suppression

1 Come onto the floor and lie down on your back ensuring there is at least two feet of space behind you. Come into Shoulder Stand.

2 Exhale and begin to bend from your hips, gradually lowering both feet behind you. Hips are raised and toes are resting on the floor. Keeping your legs straight, rest your arms out behind you on the floor, palms facing down. You can clasp your hands if you prefer. Lift your thighs up.

3 Take five deep breaths. Slowly roll your spine, vertebrae by vertebrae, to the floor and rest in Relaxation pose.

Modifications/Props:

• If your toes do not reach the floor, support your back with your hands as in Shoulder Stand.

• To support your shoulders to come into the pose, stack 2-3 folded blankets on top of one another. Blankets should be folded in a rectangular shape. Lie on the blankets with the tops of your shoulders resting on the edge of longer side on the blanket. The back of your head should rest on the floor.

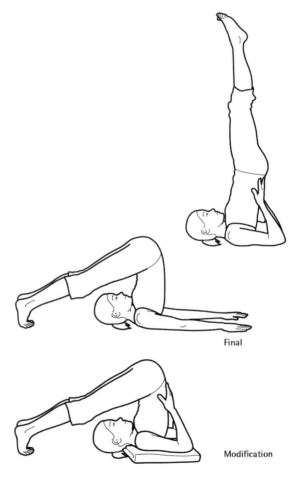

Final

Modification

Prayer Twist (Parsvakonasana)

Level: Intermediate
Posture Type: Standing, Balancing, and Twisting
Caution: Back injury and high or low blood pressure
Recommended: Loss of Appetite

1 Stand tall in Mountain pose. Hands in prayer position in front of your sternum.

2 Exhale, bend your knees into a squat. Knees and feet are together. Make sure you can see your toes.

3 Inhale and exhale, keep your hands in prayer position and bring your left elbow to the outside of your right thigh. Continue bending your left elbow, bringing your left palm to face the ceiling. Keep your right palm on top of your left palm. Hips dip low. Lengthen the twist by bringing your chest forward and your buttocks back.

4 Take five deep breaths. When you are ready to come out of the pose, exhale and return to Mountain pose. Repeat on the other side.

Modifications/Props:

• If you need balance support, rest your sacrum on a wall when lowering your body into a squatting position.

• If it is difficult to hold this pose while standing, come into the pose by lowering your body to squat in a chair.

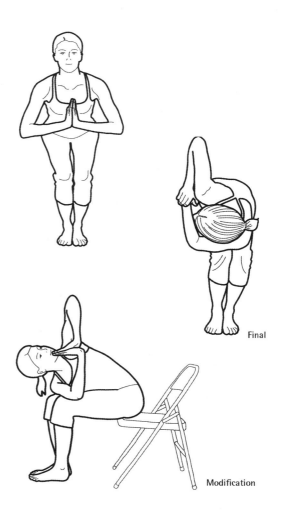

Final

Modification

Relaxation Pose (Savasana)

Level: Beginner
Posture Type: Restorative
Caution: None
Recommended: Anxiety & Stress, Chemo Brain, Constipation, Depression, Diarrhea, Fatigue, Headaches, Hot Flashes, Immune Suppression, Insomnia, Loss of Appetite, Loss of Libido, Lymphedema, Nausea & Vomiting, Pain, Peripheral Neuropathy, Shortness of Breath, Urinary Retention & Incontinence

1 Come onto the floor. Lie comfortably on your back with your legs extended evenly from your waist. Feet are hip-width apart. Allow your toes to fall softly out to the sides. Gently close your eyes. Lips are relaxed.

2 Inhale, separate your arms so your hands are about 45 degrees from your body with palms facing up. Hands are relaxed.

3 Exhale, let go of all of your tension and relax your whole body. Soften your face and relax your mind and thoughts. Concentrate fully on your breath.

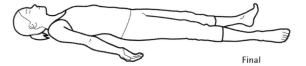

Final

4 Begin deep breathing. Stay in this pose for 5-15 minutes. When you are ready to come out of the pose, gently roll to your side, preferably your right side, and take three deep breaths. Exhale, press your hands against the floor to push yourself up into a seated position. Head comes up last.

Modifications/Props:

• To make the pose more restorative, place a folded blanket or pillow under your head and neck, shoulders, lower back, and feet. Cover yourself with a blanket.

Revolving Side Angle Pose
(Parivrtta Parsvakonasana)

Level: Intermediate
Posture Type: Standing, Balancing, and Twisting
Caution: Back injury and high or low blood pressure
Contraindication: Neck injury
Recommended: Anxiety & Stress, Constipation, Depression, Fatigue, Immune Suppression

1 Stand tall in Mountain pose.

2 Exhale, bend your knees, and step your right foot out 3-5 feet from your left. Turn your right foot out about 90 degrees and turn your left foot slightly inwards to a 45 degree angle. Align your right heel in a direct line to the arch of your left foot.

3 Inhale, bring your arms out and parallel to the floor.

4 Exhale, turn your hips to the right so that your hips are in line with your right foot.

5 Inhale and exhale, bend your right knee. Right thigh is parallel to the floor.

6 Inhale and exhale, twisting to the right, lean your upper body down and bring your left hand to the outside or inside of your right foot.

7 Inhale and exhale, extend your right arm up to your right ear and slide your shoulder blades down your back. Keep your neck long and tuck in your chin. Avoid arching your spine.

8 Take five deep breaths. Gently look up toward the inside of your right upper arm. When you are ready to come out of the pose, inhale, press into your left heel and slowly come back to the starting position. Repeat on the other side.

Modifications/Props:

• If you need balance support, stand with your back heel against a wall. Rather than extending your top arm, place the hand of your top arm on your hip.

• If you are unable to reach the floor with your palm or fingertips, place your supporting hand on a block placed either next to your inner or outer foot.

• If your neck feels tense, keep your head in a neutral position or look down at the floor.

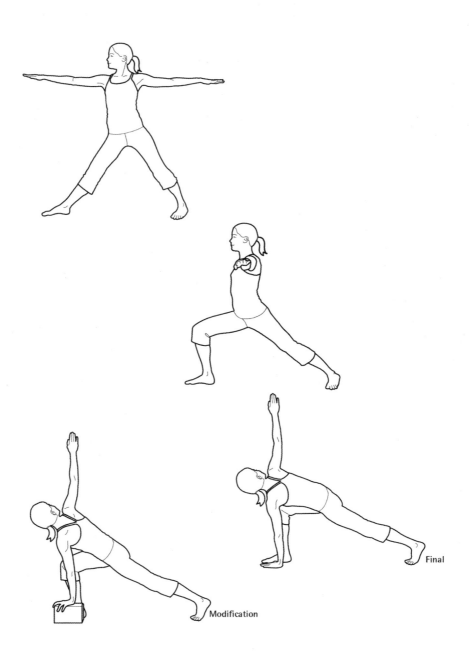

Modification

Final

Seated Forward Bend
(Paschimottanasana)

Level: Beginner
Posture Type: Seated
Caution: Back injury
Recommended: Loss of Appetite, Lymphedema, Urinary Retention &
Incontinence

1 Come onto the floor. Sit up tall with your legs straight out in front of you. Feet are together and hands are flat on the floor, just behind your hips. Fingertips are pointing forward.

2 Inhale, extend through your spine, lift your chin and raise your arms above you.

3 Exhale, reach forward from your hips, not your waist. Try to grab your ankles or feet or bring your thumb and index finger to hook onto your big toes.

4 Inhale, lengthen your spine and look up.

5 Exhale, use your arms to draw yourself forward over your legs. Bend your elbows out to the sides as you extend your chin toward your shins.

6 Take 5-10 deep breaths. With each inhalation lengthen your upper body and with each exhalation extend into the forward bend. Look at your toes. When you are ready to come out of the pose, inhale, lift your chest off your thighs by raising and extending your arms and come back to a neutral sitting position.

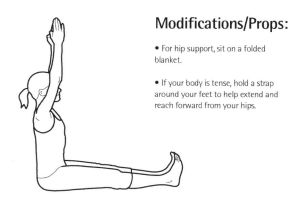

Modifications/Props:

• For hip support, sit on a folded blanket.

• If your body is tense, hold a strap around your feet to help extend and reach forward from your hips.

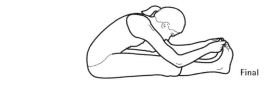

Final

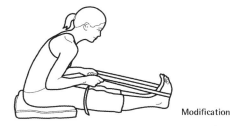

Modification

Shoulderstand (Sarvangasana)

Level: Advanced
Posture Type: Inversion
Caution: Neck injury, high or low blood pressure, dizziness, lymphedema, and pregnancy (unless experienced with this pose)
Recommended: Constipation, Depression, Hot Flashes, Immune Suppression, Urinary Retention & Incontinence

1 Come to the floor. Lie comfortably on your back with your feet together. Bring your arms alongside your body with palms facing down.

2 Inhale, pressing your arms into the floor, lift your legs up away from the floor so that your knees come toward your face. Bend your elbows and bring your hands to your lower back. Walk your hands towards your shoulder blades and spread your palms.

3 When you feel stable, inhale and straighten your legs to a 90 degree angle to the floor, drawing your belly in to support your back. Continue to press your upper arms and shoulders into the floor. Look toward the tip of your nose.

4 Take 5-20 deep breaths. When you are ready to come out of the pose, exhale and bend your knees into your chest or bring your feet towards the floor behind you. Bring your arms alongside your body with palms facing down. Slowly roll your spine, vertebrae by vertebrae, to the floor and rest in Relaxation pose.

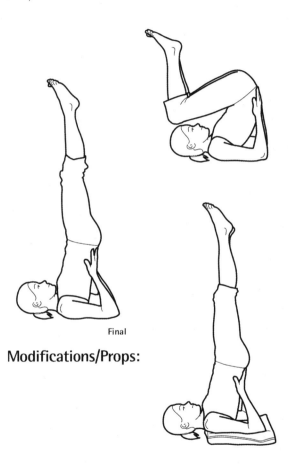

Final

Modifications/Props:

Modification

Standing Forward Bend
(Uttanasana)

Level: Intermediate
Posture Type: Standing
Caution: Back injury, dizziness, and high or low blood pressure
Recommended: Chemo Brain, Constipation, Depression, Fatigue, Insomnia, Nausea and Vomiting, Urinary Retention & Incontinence

1 Stand tall in Mountain pose, bringing your hands to your hips.

2 Exhale, bend forward from your hips, bringing your forehead toward your knees, and press your palms down into the floor or hold where comfortable. Fingertips are in line with your toes. Bend your knees if needed.

3 Take 5-10 deep breaths. With each inhalation lengthen your upper body and with each exhalation extend into the forward bend. Look at your toes. When you are ready to come out of the pose, bring your hands to your hips. Inhale, lift your chest forward and come back to stand in Mountain pose.

Modifications/Props:

• If you have any back injuries, come into the posture with your knees bent.

• If you need balance support, stand with your back against a wall.

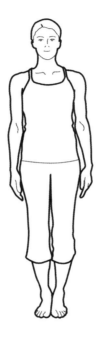

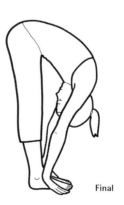

Final

Standing Head to Knee Pose
(Dandayamana Janushirasana)

Level: Intermediate
Posture Type: Standing and Balancing
Caution: High or low blood pressure
Contraindication: Knee injury and ankle injury
Recommended: Peripheral Neuropathy

1 Stand tall in Mountain pose.

2 Inhale, shifting your weight onto your left foot, bring your right foot off the floor. Grabbing the sole of your right foot with both hands, interlace your hands under the arch of your foot. Contract your left thigh, being careful not to lock your knee, to keep the standing leg straight and strong. Shift the weight in your left leg slightly forward.

3 Exhale, slowly pushing your right foot up, extend your right leg out and parallel to the floor.

4 Inhale, lengthen your spine.

5 Exhale, pulling your belly into your spine, extend your upper body forward from the hips. Lower your head to your right knee and tuck your chin into your chest.

6 Take three deep breaths. Inhale, slowly come up and place your right foot on the floor. Stand in Mountain pose. Repeat on the other side.

Modifications/Props:

• If you need balance support, stand with your back against a wall.

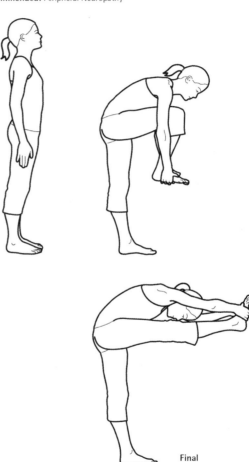

Final

Straight Leg Seated Spinal Twist
(Matsyendrasana)

Level: Beginner
Posture Type: Seated and Twisting
Caution: Back injury and neck injury
Recommended: Anxiety, Fatigue, Immune Suppression, Peripheral Neuropathy, Urinary Retention & Incontinence

1 Come onto the floor. Sit up tall with your legs straight out in front of you.

2 Exhale, cross your right foot over your left knee, placing it flat on the floor on the outside of your lower left thigh. Place your right hand behind you for support.

3 Inhale, bring your left arm up towards the ceiling.

4 Exhale, bring your left arm around the outside of your right knee, bending at the elbow.

5 Inhale, lengthen your sacrum into the floor.

6 Exhale, gently rotate your chest and head to the right. Look over your right shoulder.

7 Take five deep breaths. With each inhalation lengthen your upper body and with each exhalation twist a little more. When you are ready to come out of the pose, exhale and slowly come back to the starting position. Repeat on the other side.

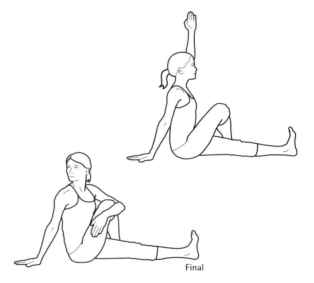

Final

Modifications/Props:

• For hip support, sit on a folded blanket.

• If it is difficult to sit on the floor with your legs straight out in front of you, come into the pose sitting in a chair. Bring your left hand to your right knee. Extend your right arm behind you and gently rotate your chest and head to the right. Repeat on the other side.

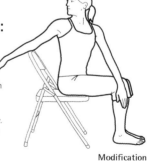

Modification

Supine Knee Squeeze
(Pavanmuktasana)

Level: Beginner
Posture Type: Restorative
Caution: Pregnancy and neck injury
Recommended: Constipation, Urinary Retention & Incontinence

1 Come onto the floor. Lie comfortably on your back with your knees bent and feet flat on the floor.

2 Exhale, bring both of your knees up to your chest. Wrap your hands around the top part of your shins or underneath your knees and clasp your hands together. Keep your lower back on the floor.

3 Take five deep breaths. For an additional massage to your back, gently roll side to side while holding your knees to your chest. Inhale, gently bring your chin to your knees and hold for one deep breath.

4 Exhale, release and rest in Relaxation pose.

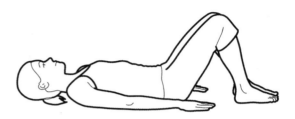

Modifications/Props:

• If your neck is tense, do not bring your chin to your knees.

• If you need back and knee support, place a pillow under your knees and wrap your hands on the top part of your shins.

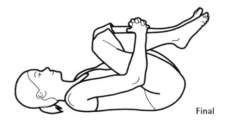

Final

Supine Twist
(Supta Matsyendrasana)

Level: Beginner
Posture Type: Twisting
Caution: Back injury and neck injury
Recommended: Constipation, Fatigue, Urinary Retention & Incontinence

1 Come onto the floor. Lie comfortably on your back with your knees bent and feet flat on the floor.

2 Inhale, bring your right knee toward your chest and extend your left leg out straight.

3 Exhale, twisting from the waist, bring your right knee across the left side of your body. With your left hand on your outer right knee, rest your knee on the floor. Keep your left leg straight and both shoulders on the floor. Extend your right arm out to your right side. Turn your neck and head to the right.

4 Take 5-10 deep breaths. When you are ready to come out of the pose, exhale and slowly come back to the starting position. Repeat on the other side.

Modifications/Props:

• If your neck is tense, do not turn your neck and head.

• If your knees do not reach the floor or if you want to make this pose more restorative, place a folded blanket under your arms and knees.

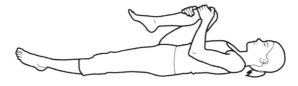

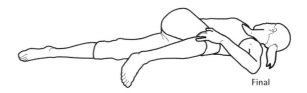

Final

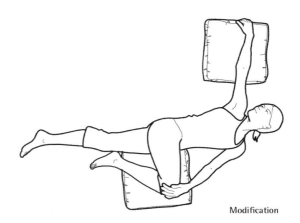

Modification

Tree Pose (Vrksasana)

Level: Beginner
Posture Type: Standing and Balancing
Caution: Knee injury and high or low blood pressure
Recommended: Anxiety & Stress, Depression, Insomnia, Peripheral Neuropathy

1 Stand tall in Mountain pose. Shifting your weight onto your left foot, bend your right knee and bring your right heel to rest on the inside of your left ankle.

2 Inhale, lift your right leg with the help of your hands.

3 Exhale, place the sole of your right foot against the inner part of your left thigh.

4 Inhale, bring your arms out to your sides and in line with your shoulders.

5 Exhale, bring your hands together in prayer position in front of your sternum.

6 Take five deep breaths, focusing your attention on your inhalation and exhalation. Look at a point on the floor in front of you. When you are ready to come out of the pose, exhale and straighten your right leg back down to the floor. Relax your hands at your sides and come to stand in Mountain pose. Repeat on the other side.

Modifications/Props:

• If you are unable to lift your leg so that your foot rests against the inner part of your thigh, rest your foot on your calf or ankle.

• If you need balance support, stand with your back against a wall.

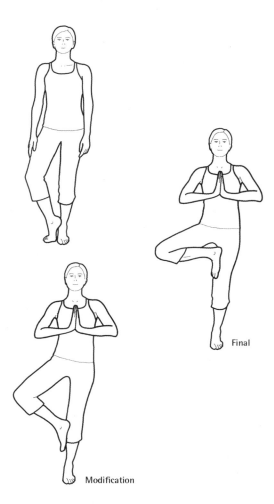

Final

Modification

Triangle Pose (Trikonasana)

Level: Intermediate
Posture Type: Standing and Balancing
Caution: Back injury and high or low blood pressure
Contraindication: Neck injury
Recommended: Constipation, Depression, Immune Suppression, Lymphedema, Peripheral Neuropathy

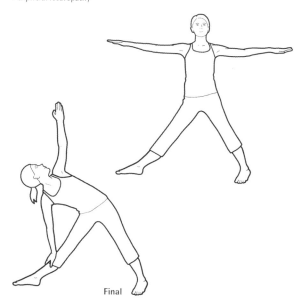

1 Stand tall in Mountain pose.

2 Exhale, slightly bend your knees, and step your right foot out 3-5 feet from your left foot. Turn your right foot out about 90 degrees and turn your left foot slightly inwards to a 45 degree angle. Align your right heel in a direct line to the arch of your left foot.

3 Inhale, bring your arms out and parallel to the floor.

4 Exhale, bending from your hips, extend your upper body over your right thigh.

5 Inhale, sliding your right hand down your thigh, place your right hand on your shin and rotate your upper body to the left.

6 Exhale, extend your left arm up to the ceiling and slide your shoulder blades down your back. Keep your neck long and tuck in your chin. The side of your upper body is parallel to the floor. Avoid arching your spine.

7 Take five deep breaths. Gently look up toward your left hand. When you are ready to come out of the pose, inhale, press into your left heel and slowly come back to the starting position. Repeat on the other side.

Final

Modifications/Props:

• If you need balance support, stand with your back against a wall. Rather than extending your top arm, place the hand of your top arm on your hip.

• If you are unable to reach the floor with your palm or fingertips, place your supporting hand on a block.

• If your neck feels tense, keep your head in a neutral position.

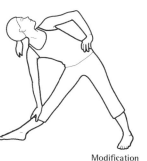

Modification

Twisting Triangle Pose
(Parivrtta Trikonasana)

Level: Intermediate
Posture Type: Standing, Balancing, and Twisting
Caution: Back injury and high or low blood pressure
Contraindication: Neck injury
Recommended: Anxiety & Stress, Constipation, Depression, Fatigue, Immune Suppression, Lymphedema

1 Stand tall in Mountain pose.

2 Exhale, bend your knees, and step your right foot out 3-5 feet from your left foot. Turn your right foot out about 90 degrees and turn your left foot slightly inwards to a 45 degree angle. Align your right heel in a direct line to the arch of your left foot.

3 Inhale, bring your arms out and parallel to the floor.

4 Exhale, turn your hips to the right so that your hips are in line with your right foot.

5 Inhale and exhale, bringing your left hand to the outside or inside of your right foot.

6 Inhale, slightly lower your left hip.

7 Exhale, extend your right arm up to the ceiling and slide your shoulder blades down your back. Keep your neck long and tuck in your chin. Avoid arching your spine.

8 Take five deep breaths. Gently look up toward your right hand. When you are ready to come out of the pose, inhale, press into your left heel and slowly come back to the starting position. Repeat on the other side.

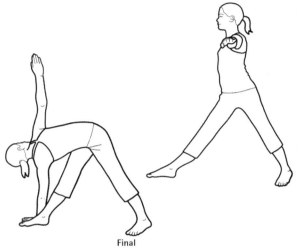

Final

Modifications/Props:

• If you need balance support, stand with your back heel against a wall. Rather than extending your top arm, place the hand of your top arm on your hip.

• If you are unable to reach the floor with your palm or fingertips, place your supporting hand on your shin or on a block placed either next to your inner or outer foot.

• If your neck feels tense, keep your head in a neutral position or look down at the floor.

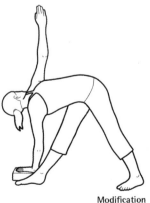

Modification

Wheel Pose
(Urdhva Dhanurasana)

Level: Advanced
Posture Type: Backbend
Caution: Carpal tunnel syndrome, pregnancy, and high or low blood pressure
Contraindication: Neck injury
Recommended: Anxiety & Stress, Depression, Fatigue, Immune Suppression, Shortness of Breath

1 Come onto the floor. Lie comfortably on your back with your knees bent and feet flat on the floor. Feet are hip-width apart and heels are close to your buttocks.

2 Inhale, place your palms down next to your ears. Fingertips pointing toward your shoulders. Pull your elbows in to align with your shoulders and slide your shoulder blades down your back.

3 Exhale, press your hips, buttocks, and then crown of your head off the floor as you push your arms and legs down into the floor. Elbows straighten and thighs are stretched. Keep your back and head relaxed and your thighs parallel and hip-width apart.

4 Take five deep breaths. Look at the wall behind you. When you are ready to come out of the pose, exhale and slowly release. Bring your knees to your chest.

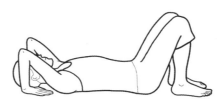

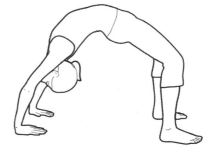

Final

Modifications/Props:

• If you are unable to come into the pose, modify the pose by coming into Bridge pose.

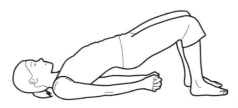

Modification

Appendix E
Glycemic Index

The Glycemic Index (GI) describes the type of carbohydrate in foods and its potential to raise blood glucose and insulin levels. Blood glucose levels are determined by both the quality and quantity of carbohydrate. Therefore, it is important to have sensible food portions when following a low glycemic diet. Foods with a low GI value cause smaller fluctuations in blood glucose and insulin levels.

The table below categorizes foods based on the GI of the food. A high glycemic index is considered to be between 70 and 100. High GI foods should be avoided or consumed rarely. Foods with a moderate GI value fall between 55 and 70. Foods with a GI value below 55 are foods with a low GI and should be emphasized every day. Serving sizes should follow the recommended guidelines (Appendix G).

Food Category	Foods to Avoid/ Eat Rarely GI > 70	Foods to Eat Weekly GI 55 to 70	Foods to Eat Daily GI ≤ 55
Breads/ Grains/ Cereals/ Pasta	White bread, French bread, couscous, basmati, gnocchi, macaroni & cheese, sugared/frosted cereals, muffins, granola, rice cakes, bagels, saltine crackers, doughnuts	Brown rice, white rice, millet, wheat, spaghetti (cooked al dente), pita bread, capellini, instant noodles, macaroni, ravioli, tortellini, oatmeal	Rye, 100% wholegrain breads, pumpernickel, pearled barley, quinoa, fettuccine, bulgur, vermicelli, spaghetti (protein enriched), muesli, biscuits made with dried fruit/whole grains and/or oats, muffins made with dried fruit and/or nuts, whole grains and oats, whole grain cereals with at least 4–5 grams of fiber/ serving
Vegetables	Potatoes, carrots, parsnips, pumpkin, beets, French fries, rutabaga	Green peas, corn, sweet potato, yams, beats	Broccoli, Brussels sprouts, kale, asparagus, cabbage, okra, turnips, mushrooms, spinach, tomato, zucchini, cauliflower, celery, cucumber, green beans, green pepper, salads (emphasize dark colored leaves; avoid iceberg), Bok Choy, mustard greens

(Continued)

(*Continued*)

Food Category	Foods to Avoid/ Eat Rarely GI > 70	Foods to Eat Weekly GI 55 to 70	Foods to Eat Daily GI ≤ 55
Fruits	Watermelon, papaya, cantaloupe, honeydew	Banana, kiwi, mango, grapes, pineapple, raisins	Apples, fresh or dried apricots, cherries, grapefruit, orange, peach, pear, plum, raspberries, strawberries, blueberries, figs
Legumes/ Beans	None	None	All legumes should be emphasized, including bean-based products such as tempeh, tofu, and hummus
Meat/Fish/ Poultry/ Dairy	Fried meat/fish/ poultry, cheese spreads, hot dogs, fast food sandwiches	Lean beef burger, chicken burger, veggie burger	Scrambled or hard-boiled eggs, cottage cheese, cheese, game (duck, peasant), canned tuna or salmon, Low fat/ non-sweetened yogurt, skim milk, whole milk, cheese (choose low-fat varieties)
Snacks	Pretzels, fast food products, packaged sweets, chips, rice cakes	Chocolate (cocoa chocolate only), popcorn, oatmeal cookies, angel food cake	Nuts/seeds (Brazil nuts, almonds, sesame seeds, almonds, walnuts, hazelnuts, pumpkin seeds), dips (hummus, guacamole, or any bean-based spread), edamame (soybeans)
Condiments	Mayonnaise, butter	Honey, table sugar, mustard	Olive oil, Agave nectar (sweetener)
Beverages	Soda, sweetened juices	Fresh, non-sweetened juice (apple, orange)	Tea (no sugar), soy milk, sparkling or flat water

Simple Food Substitutions May Also Help You Follow a Low GI Diet

- Use breakfast cereals based on oats, barley and bran
- Use breads with whole grains, stone-ground flour, sour dough
- Reduce the amount of potatoes you eat
- Replace high GI with low GI fruits and vegetables
- Use Basmati or Doongara rice also known as "smart rice"

- Choose whole-grain rice, Kashi, or quinoa
- Eat plenty of salad vegetables with a vinaigrette dressing

There are many books and websites that may be referred to for information on a specific food items. Below are some good references:

- http://www.glycemicindex.com/. This website contains a unique glycemic index database that provides a search engine where you can input in a food item and it will provide the glycemic index including serving size.
- http://www.hsph.harvard.edu/nutritionsource/what-should-you-eat/carbohydrates-full-story/ from the Harvard School of Public Health. Provides information on the glycemic index.

Appendix F
High Fiber Food Sources

Fiber can be found in a variety of foods such as vegetables, fruits, whole grains, beans and legumes. There are two types of fiber, soluble and insoluble, and they have different functions.

Soluble fiber
• Attracts water, slowing down the food passing through your intestines. May reduce the symptoms of diarrhea.
• Makes you feel fuller for a longer time, and may help in weight management.
• When food is digested slowly, blood glucose levels do not rise as quickly, so soluble fiber might benefit people with diabetes in controlling blood sugar.
• Soluble fiber can also lower cholesterol levels and lower risk for certain conditions such as heart disease when eaten regularly as part of a healthy diet.

Insoluble fiber
• Tends to "flush out" your system, good for removing toxic substances in your body.
• A diet high in insoluble fiber, together with plenty of fluids, can regulate bowel movements and help reduce constipation.

Recommended fiber intakes per day

Age	Recommended fiber intake (grams) for women	Recommended fiber intake (grams) for males
1–3	19	19
4–8	25	25
9–13	26	31
14–18	26	38
19–50	25	38
50 and above	21	30
Pregnancy & Lactation		
Pregnancy	28	
Lactation	29	

High fiber foods

Food	Serving Size	Total Fiber (g)	Soluble Fiber (g)	Insoluble Fiber (g)
Fruit				
Figs, dried	3 medium	10.5	4.9	5.6
Raspberries	1 cup	8	2.1	5.9
Blackberries	1 cup	7.6	1.9	5.7
Pear with skin	1 medium	5.1	1.9	3.2
Tangerine	2 medium	5	4.4	0.6
Cranberries	1 cup	5	1.7	3.3
Orange	1 large	4	2.5	1.5
Apricot, whole	5	4	2.1	1.9
Red apple with skin	1 medium	4	1.4	2.6
Mangoes	1 medium	3.7	2.2	1.5
Blueberries	1 cup	3.5	0.7	2.8
Strawberries	1 cup	3.4	1.3	2.1
Bananas	1 banana	3.1	0.8	2.3
Prunes	5 small	3	1.8	1.2
Vegetables				
Cooked spinach	1 cup	7	2.2	4.8
Cooked Brussels sprouts	1 cup	6.4	3.4	3
Red cabbage, cooked	2 cups	6	0.3	5.7
Acorn squash, baked	1 cup	6	0.7	5.3
butternut squash, baked	1 cup	5.7	2.3	3.4
Parsnips	1 cup	5.4	2.7	2.7
Collard greens, cooked	1 cup	5.3	2.4	2.9
Okra	1 cup	5.2	1.3	3.9
Cooked broccoli	1 cup	5	2.5	2.5
Cooked turnip greens	1 cup	5	1.6	3.4
Cauliflower	1 cup	4.9	2	2.9
Tomato sauce, puree	1 cup	4.8	2.3	2.5
White potato, baked w/ skin	1 medium	4.8	2	2.8
Sweet potato with skin	1 medium	4.8	1.8	3
Cooked carrots	1 cup	4.7	2.6	2.1
Artichoke hearts, canned/jar	4 small	4.5	3.3	1.2
Green peas	1/2 cup	4.4	1.3	3.1
Cooked beets	1 cup	4	1.8	2.2

(*Continued*)

(Continued)

Food	Serving Size	Total Fiber (g)	Soluble Fiber (g)	Insoluble Fiber (g)
Cooked green beans	1 cup	4	1.6	2.4
Mushrooms	1 cup	3.4	0.4	3
Peppers, sweet, raw	1 cup	3.1	1.3	1.8
Raw carrots	1 cup	3.1	1.5	1.6
Cooked cabbage	1 cup	2.9	1.2	1.7
Eggplant, cooked	1 cup	2.5	0.8	1.7
Beans/Legumes				
Navy beans, cooked	1/2 cup	9.6	3.2	6.4
Split peas, cooked	1/2 cup	8	2.5	5.5
Lentils, cooked	1/2 cup	7.8	0.9	6.9
Pinto beans, cooked	1/2 cup	7.7	1.8	5.9
Black beans, cooked	1/2 cup	7.5	3	4.5
Kidney beans, cooked	1/2 cup	6.9	2	4.9
Lima (butter) beans	1/2 cup	6.6	1.7	4.9
Chickpeas, cooked	1/2 cup	6.3	1.9	4.4
Soy beans	1/2 cup	5.2	2.3	2.9
Baked beans, canned	1/2 cup	5.2	2.6	2.6
Bread/Cereals/Grains				
Fiber One cereal	1/2 cup	11.9	0.8	11.1
All-Bran cereal	1/2 cup	8.8	1.4	7.4
Raisin Bran cereal	1 cup	6.8	1.2	4.6
Pearl Barley, cooked	1 cup	6	1.6	4.4
Grape Nuts cereal	1/2 cup	5	1.6	3.4
Bulgur, cooked	1/2 cup	4.1	0.7	3.4
Whole-wheat bread	2 slices	4	0.8	3.2
Shredded wheat, spoon size	1/2 cup	4	0.5	3.5
Oatmeal, cooked	1 cup	4	2.1	1.9
Rye bread	2 slices	3	1.6	1.4
Cheerios	1 cup	3	1.4	1.6
Oat bran, cooked	1/2 cup	2.7	1.5	1.2
Seeds/Nuts				
Sunflower seed kernels (dry roasted, w/ salt added)	1/2 cup	6	2.4	3.6
Peanuts, dry roasted	1/4 cup	4.6	1.5	3.1
Almonds, sliced	1/4 cup	3.5	0.6	2.9

Source: USDA nutrient database

Appendix G
Managing Food Portions

1. In some cases, half is better than whole. Instead of getting rid of all the foods you like, decrease the portion size by half and supplement your meal with veggies, salad or a light soup. For instance, eat half a sandwich for lunch with carrots and some nuts.

2. Your plate should visually look like this →

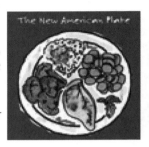

— At least 2/3rds of the plate should be vegetables, fruits, whole grains, and/or beans. One third or less should be animal protein, preferably lean meats like chicken or fish.

The New American Plate. American Institute of Cancer Research. http://www.aicr.org/

3. Slim down that dinner! When dining out, share your entrée with someone. Alternatively, immediately ask for half of your meal in a to-go container. If you package half of your food at the beginning of your meal chances are you won't open that container and eat the rest of it until later.

4. Choose an appetizer or salad as your main entrée instead of a full course.

5. *Out of sight, out of mind.* Ask the waiter to avoid bringing the bread basket or other luring concoctions.

6. Plan ahead. Carry healthy snacks with you to reduce the temptation to "grab and go" when you are hungry. Measure out a small portion of your snack and avoid carrying the whole bag. Either buy individual bags one at a time, or divide the big bag into single serving snack bags. Healthy snack items: whole wheat crackers, dried fruit, carrot sticks, fresh fruit, pretzels, edamame, and homemade trail mix (nuts and dried fruit).

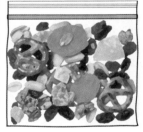

7. Evaluate your servings. Check the box and learn what a controlled portion of your favorite snacks look like by measuring them out the next time you eat them.

8. Say NO to super sized food items.

9. If you are at a buffet or a family style restaurant, fill your plate once or fill half your plate if you go up several times. It is incredibly challenging to eat sensible portions when attacked by the phrase "all-you-can-eat;" if possible, avoid these places entirely.

10. Cook Once, Eat Twice. Think ahead and break your leftovers down into individually-sized containers so that when you reach into the fridge, you'll be retrieving just enough for one helping.

11. At home, serve yourself ONCE and keep seconds out of sight. After serving yourself keep food away from the table where it's all too easy to go for seconds. If you give yourself a second to wait out the urge, you will find that you weren't that hungry after all. So, take a deep breath and remember: it takes about 15 to 20 minutes to feel satiated.

12. Even when you are hungry, chew each mouthful of food properly, at least 10 times before swallowing. Eating slower helps you pay attention to your stomach and stop when you feel full.

13. Learn the basic serving standards when dining out or making your own meals. Here's a guide to help you know what a serving size looks like:

Type of Food	Serving Size	Serving Size Visual
GRAINS		
Dry Cereal Flakes	1 cup	
Cooked Cereal, Rice, Pasta or Potato; Pretzels, Crackers	1/2 cup	
VEGETABLES AND FRUIT		
Raw Leafy Vegetables	1 cup	
Other Vegetables, Cooked, Raw and/or Chopped; Chopped Fruit; Beans, Legumes	1/2 cup	
Whole Fruit (Apple, Orange, Pear); Vegetable or Fruit Juice	1 cup	

(*Continued*)

(*Continued*)

Type of Food	Serving Size	Serving Size Visual
DAIRY		
Cheese	1 oz	
Milk or Yogurt	1 cup	
MEAT AND OTHERS		
Meat, Fish and Poultry	3 oz	
Oils (olive, canola, flax), Nut Butters (almond, cashew, peanut), Cream Cheese, Butter	1 TBS	
Nuts, Seeds, or Dried Fruit	1 oz	

Appendix H
References

Bensky, D., Clavey, S., & Stoger, E. (2006). *Chinese Herbal Medicine Materia Medica* (3rd ed. revised). Seattle, WA: Eastland Press.

Borud, E.K., Alraek, T., White, A., Fonnebo, V., Eggen, A.E., Hammar, M., *et al.* (2009). The Acupuncture on Hot Flushes Among Menopausal Women (ACUFLASH) Study, a Randomized Controlled Trial. *Menopause,* 16, 484–93.

Byers, D.C. (1983). *Better Health with Foot Reflexology: The Ingham Method of Reflexology.* Saint Petersburg, FL: Ingham Publishing Inc.

Deadman, P., Al-Khafaji, M., & Baker, K. (1998). *A Manual of Acupuncture.* East Sussex, England: Journal of Chinese Medicine Publications.

Ergil, M.C., & Ergil, K.V. (2009). *Pocket Atlas of Chinese Medicine.* Stuttgart, Germany: Thieme Publications.

Essential Oil Desk Reference (4th ed.). (2009). Orem, UT: Essential Science Publishing.

Field, Derek. (1994). *Anatomy: Palpation and Surface Markings.* Oxford, England: Butterworth-Heinemann.

Finando, D., & Finando, S. (1999). *Informed Touch: A Clinician's Guide to the Evaluation and Treatment of Myofascial Disorders.* Rochester, VT: Healing Arts Press.

Fritz, S. (2003). *Mosby's Fundamentals of Therapeutic Massage* (3rd ed.). St. Louis, MO: Mosby.

Gawain, S. (2002). *Creative Visualization: Use the Power of Your Imagination to Create What You Want In Your Life.* Novato, CA: Nataraj Publishing.

Hervik, J., & Mjåland, O. (2009). Acupuncture for the Treatment of Hot Flashes in Breast Cancer Patients, a Randomized, Controlled Trial. *Breast Cancer Research and Treatment,* 116, 311–6.

Hughes, D., Ladas, E., Rooney, D., & Kelly, K. (2008). Massage Therapy as a Supportive Care Intervention for Children with Cancer. *Oncology Nursing Forum,* 35, 431–42.

Iyengar, B.K.S. (2001). *Yoga: The Path to Holistic Health.* London, England: Dorling Kindersley.

Kuntz, B., & Kunz, K. (2006). *Hand Reflexology.* New York, NY: DK Publishing.

Kuntz, B., & Kunz, K. (2005). *The Complete Guide to Foot Reflexology* (3rd ed.). Albuquerque, NM: RRP Press.

People's Desk Reference for Essential Oils. (1999). Orem, UT: Essential Science Publishing.

Singles Therapeutic Essential Oil Guide: A Companion Guide to the World of Therapeutic Essential Oils. (2001). Petaluma, CA: Oshadi.

Tortora, G., & Anagnostakos, N. (1981). *Principles of Anatomy and Physiology.* New York, NY: Harper & Row Publishers.

Travell, J., & Simons, D. (1983). *Myofascial Pain and Dysfunction: The Trigger Point Manual Vol I. Upper Half of Body.* Baltimore, MD: Lippincott Williams & Wilkins.

Travell, J., & Simons, D. (1992). *Myofascial Pain and Dysfunction: The Trigger Point Manual Vol II. The Lower Extremities.* Baltimore, MD: Lippincott Williams & Wilkins.

Ullman, D. (2010). *Homeopathic Family Medicine: Connecting Research to Quality Homeopathic Care.* Berkeley, CA: Homeopathic Educational Services.

Yoga Journal. Website: www.yogajournal.com.

Appendix I
Resources

Aromatherapy
The National Association for Holistic Aromatherapy
P.O. Box 1868
Banner Elk, NC 28604
Phone: 828-898-6161
Fax: 828-898-1965
Email: info@naha.org
Website: www.naha.org

People's Desk Reference for Essential Oils. (1999). Orem, UT: Essential Science Publishing.

Essential Oil Desk Reference (4th ed.). (2009). Orem, UT: Essential Science Publishing.

Cancer Facts and Statistics
National Cancer Institute Office of Communications and Education
Public Inquiries Office
6116 Executive Boulevard, Suite 300
Bethesda, MD 20892
Phone: 800-422-6237
Website: www.cancer.gov

Cancer Facts and Figures
American Cancer Society, Inc.
Website: www.cancer.org/Research/CancerFactsFigures

MedlinePlus®
Website: http://medlineplus.gov

Chinese Medicine /Acupressure/Acupuncture
American Association of Acupuncture and Oriental Medicine
P.O. Box 162340
Sacramento, CA 95816
Phone: 866-455-7999
Website: http://www.aaaomonline.org/

National Certification Commission for Acupuncture and Oriental Medicine
76 South Laura Street, Suite 1290
Jacksonville, FL 32202
Phone: 904-598-1005
Fax: 904-598-5001
Email: info@nccaom.org
Website: www.nccaom.org

Deadman, P., Al-Khafaji, M., & Baker, K. (1998). *A Manual of Acupuncture.* East Sussex, England: Journal of Chinese Medicine Publications.

Kaptchuk, T. (2000). *The Web That Has No Weaver: Understanding Chinese Medicine (2nd ed.).* Chicago, IL: Contemporary Books Inc.

Herbalism

American Herbalists Guild
141 Nob Hill Road
Cheshire, CT 06410
Phone: 203-272-6731
Fax: 203-272-8550
Email: ahgoffice@earthlink.net
Website: www.americanherbalist.com

Bonnie's Herbals
Website: www.bonniesherbals.com

Natural Medicines Comprehensive Database
Therapeutic Research Faculty
Website: http://naturaldatabase.therapeuticresearch.com

Homeopathy

Council for Homeopathic Certification
PMB 187
16915 SE 272nd Street Suite #100
Covington, WA 98042
Phone: 866-242-3399
Fax: 815-366-7622
Email: chcinfo@homeopathicdirectory.com
Website: www.homeopathicdirectory.com

Integrative Medicine: Definitions and Information

The Integrative Therapies Program for Children with Cancer
Herbert Irving Child & Adolescent Oncology Center
Columbia University
161 Fort Washington, IP-7
New York, NY 10032
Phone: 212-305-7829
Fax: 212-305-5848
Website: www.integrativetherapiesprogram.org

Office of Cancer Complementary and Alternative Medicine
National Cancer Institute
U.S. National Institutes of Health
6116 Executive Blvd., Suite 609, MSC 8339
Bethesda, MD 20892
Phone: 301-435-7980
Fax: 301-480-0075
Email: ncioccam1-r@mail.nih.gov
Website: http://www.cancer.gov/cam

National Center for Complementary and Alternative Medicine
National Institutes of Health
9000 Rockville Pike
Bethesda, MD 20892
Phone: 888-644-6226
Fax: 866-464-3616
Email: info@nccam.nih.gov
Website: http://nccam.nih.gov

PDQ® Cancer Information Summaries: Complementary/Alternative Medicine; Supportive and Palliative Care
National Cancer Institute
U.S. National Institutes of Health
Website: http://www.cancer.gov/cancertopics/pdq/cam;
http://www.cancer.gov/cancertopics/pdq/supportivecare

PubMed
National Library of Medicine
National Institutes of Health
Website: http://www.ncbi.nlm.nih.gov/pubmed

Society for Integrative Oncology
www.integrativeonc.org

Massage

American Massage Therapy Association
500 Davis Street, Suite 900
Evanston, IL 60201
Phone: 877-905-2700
Fax: 847-864-5196
Email: info@amtamassage.org
Website: www.amtamassage.org

Fritz, S. (1995). *Mosby's Fundamentals of Therapeutic Massage.* St. Louis, MO: Mosby Lifeline.

Nutrition

American Institute for Cancer Research
1759 R Street NW
Washington, DC 20009
Phone: 800-843-8114
Fax: 202-328-7744
Email: aicrweb@aicr.org
Website: www.aicr.org

Healthy Monday
www.healthymonday.org

Nutrition in Cancer Care (PDQ®)
National Cancer Institute
National Institutes of Health
Website: http://www.cancer.gov/cancertopics/pdq/supportivecare/nutrition/Patient

Dietary Reference Intakes
Institute of Medicine
National Academies Press
http://www.nap.edu/

Reflexology

American Reflexology Certification Board
P.O. Box 5147
Gulfport, FL 33737
Phone: 303-933-6921
Fax: 303-904-0460
Email: info@arcb.net
Website: http://www.arcb.net

Reflexology Association of America
P.O. Box 714
Chepachet, RI 02814
Phone: 980-234-0159
Fax: 401-568-6449
Email: InfoRAA@reflexology-usa.org
Website: www.reflexology-usa.org

Kuntz, B., & Kunz, K. (2005). *The Complete Guide to Foot Reflexology (3rd ed.).* Albuquerque, NM: RRP Press.

Visual Imagery

Gawain, S. (2008). *Creative Visualization: Use the Power of Your Imagination to Create What You Want in Your Life (2nd ed.).* Novato, CA: Nataraj Publishing.

Rooney, D. (2011). *Integrative Strategies for People with Cancer: A Companion of Guided Visual Imageries* [Audio CD]. Eds. E. Ladas, & K. Kelly.

Yoga

Yoga Alliance®
1701 Clarendon Boulevard, Suite 110
Arlington, VA 22209
Phone: 888-921-9642
Fax: 571-482-3336
Website: www.yogaalliance.org

Yoga Journal
Website: www.yogajournal.com

Iyengar, B.K.S. (2001). *Yoga: The Path to Holistic Health.* London, England: Dorling Kindersley.

Appendix J
Metric Conversion Table

US Equivalent	Metric
1/2 ounce	15 milliliters
1 ounce	30 milliliters
4 ounces	120 milliliters
1 drop	1/20 milliliters
1 teaspoon	5 milliliters
1 tablespoon	15 milliliters
1 cup	250 milliliters
2.2 pounds	1 kilogram
350° Fahrenheit	175° Celsius

Index